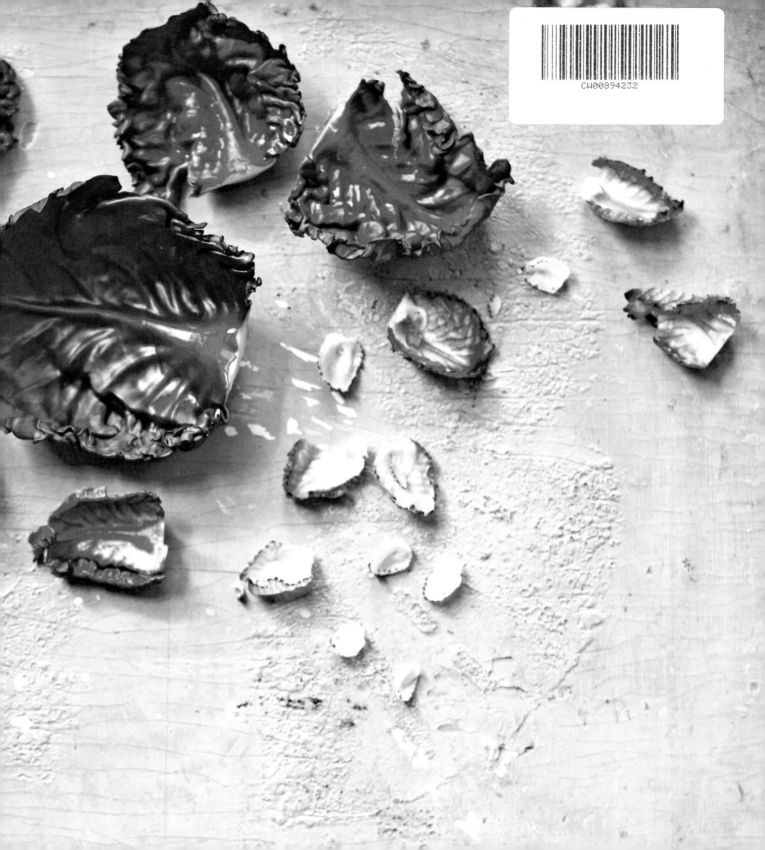

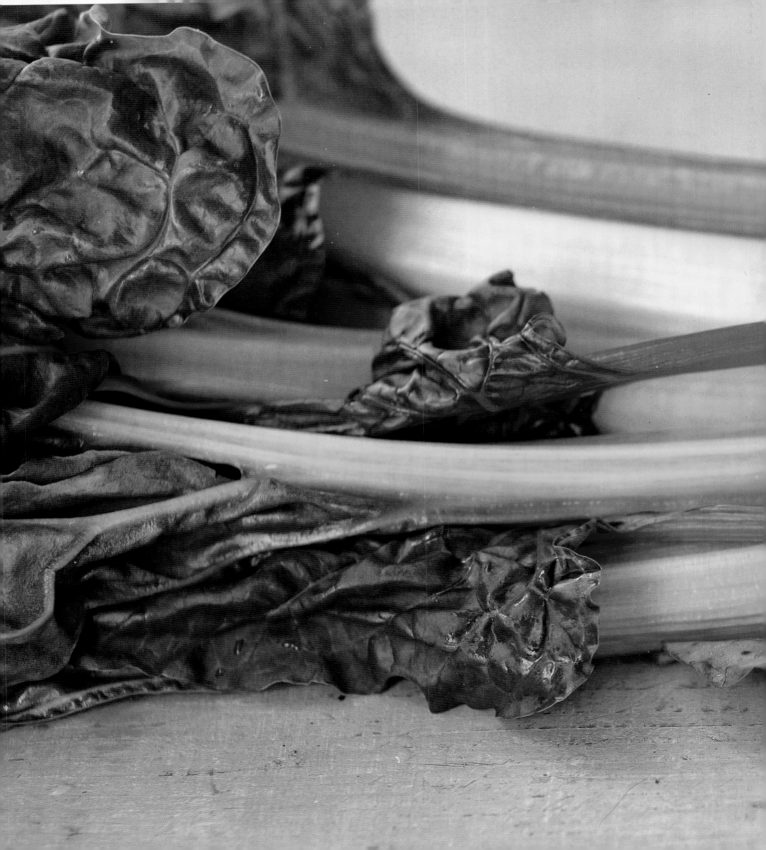

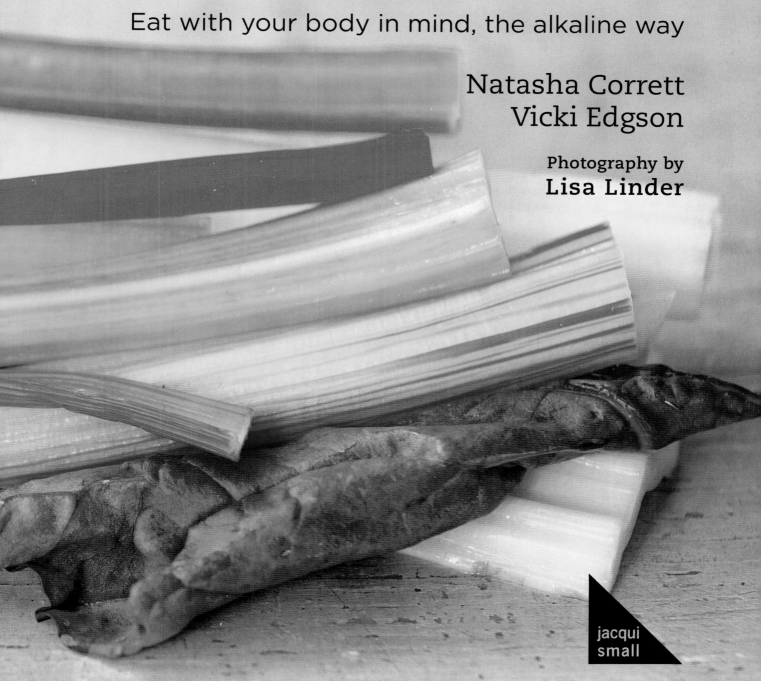

Honestly Healthy

Eat with your body in mind, the alkaline way

Natasha Corrett
Vicki Edgson

Photography by
Lisa Linder

jacqui small

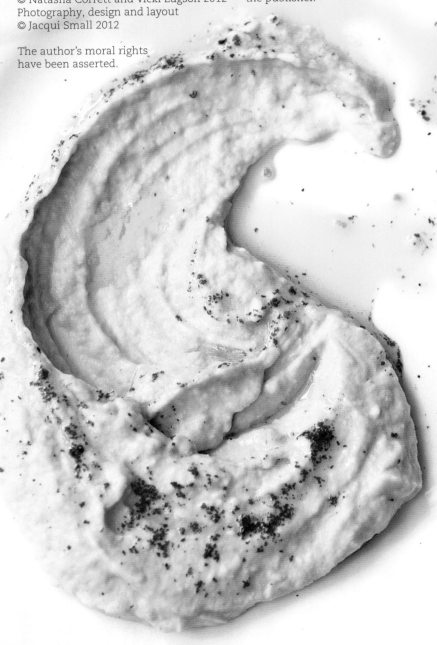

First published in 2012 by
Jacqui Small LLP
An imprint of Aurum Press
74–77 White Lion Street
London N1 9PF

Publisher: **Jacqui Small**
Managing Editor: **Kerenza Swift**
Art Director: **Penny Stock**
Photographer: **Lisa Linder**
Project Manager: **Nikki Sims**
Editor: **Jenni Davis**
Production: **Peter Colley**

ISBN: 978 1 906417 81 9

A catalogue record for this book is
available from the British Library.

2014
10

Printed in China

From Tash – I dedicate this book to
my best friend Laura who continues
to inspire me everyday and to my
Mummy and Daddy who have
supported me every step of the way.

From Vix – I dedicate this book to
my dear friend Karen, who first
made me realise how important
it is for vegetarians to better
understand how to balance their
nutrition for vital health.

When following the recipes, stick to one set
of measurements (metric, imperial or cups).
Measurements used in the recipes are
based on the following conversions:
25g = 1oz
25ml = 1fl oz
250ml = 8fl oz = 1 cup (for both liquid and
dry volume ingredients)
Note that the weight of dry ingredients
varies according to the volume so 1 cup of
flour weighs less than 1 cup of sugar.

contents

Key to symbols (see page 11)

♥♥♥ really really alkaline food or recipe

♥♥ really alkaline food or recipe

♥ alkaline food or recipe

🌱 vegan

Our Story and Passion

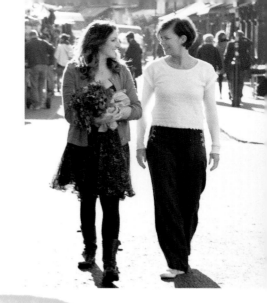

We first met on the day of Natasha's birth, when I was introduced to her as her godmother. We have, needless to say, known each other ever since. Our friendship has grown with the years, with Tash always interested to see how my career in nutrition and well-being has grown, while at the same time pursuing her own knowledge of spiritual, holistic and herbal practices alongside her passion for food – her taste buds having been influenced from an early age by her French restaurateur father.

We both share a passion for great food always starting with raw ingredients. My own mother prepared everything from scratch and I remember the best part of coming home from boarding school was always the smells wafting through from the kitchen. I now experience the same feeling every time I walk into Tash's home – there's always some delicious gluten-free cake on the table, or an extraordinary version of risotto or bean casserole.

We came together in business in May 2009, when I attended one of Tash's retreats in the deepest countryside on the Wiltshire/Dorset borders, where she had rented a large mansion for a three-day retreat. At the last minute the chef she had hired let her down and, true to form, Tash rose to the occasion and simply said, 'Then I shall have to be the chef!' She proceeded to produce some of the most fabulous vegetarian food I had ever tasted, and the weekend was a resounding success, especially at mealtimes, with everyone exclaiming just how mouthwatering the dishes were. She continued to amaze all of us as meal after meal was produced from seemingly simple ingredients – fresh, tangy, tasty and very moreish.

By the middle of the following week, over half her retreat guests had requested that Tash set up a home-delivery service, and her 'Fridge Fill' was launched – three days' worth of breakfast, lunch, dinner and snacks delivered on a Monday evening. The premise was simply that eating healthy food for at least half your week will yield improvements to your overall health and, in a matter of weeks, have you choosing more carefully when dining out, travelling on public services or just snacking from your corner store. Tash was adamant that she could start to change the eating habits of the nation by delivering really real food to a handful of people who would spread the word, organically.

'Organic where it matters' became the common thread, and before long the word had indeed spread, and Harrods invited Tash to take a selection of her produce into their store for tasting. She spent a frenetic weekend preparing dishes and painting a wooden crate with her own logo and filling it with straw, as if it had come fresh from the field and ready to serve – it looked divine, tempting and delicious!

Her presentation to Harrods was a resounding success, and she called me excitedly to tell me the news. I responded immediately with 'Do you want an investor in your business? You are clearly going places, and I would love to get involved!'

There followed much excitement, many meetings and a lot of hard work in prepping our kitchens to match up to the stringent examination procedures that any department store or supermarket deems essential, and we realised we were no longer simply preparing food for friends and clients. The commercial food industry health and safety standards are rigorous (as they should be), and there was much to learn about running our own kitchens.

Interestingly, we never did end up selling into Harrods, as Harvey Nichols and Selfridges both got wind of our brand, and made seductive moves to ply us away! We finally launched into London's Selfridges Food Hall in July 2011, with our own small refrigerated concession, and much fanfare from friends and family. News of our 'great, delicious vegetarian food' spread, and we were soon sought by many specialist food shops, stores and markets.

Tash and I both firmly stand by our brand – the importance of really real food is becoming ever more important in today's increasingly ready-prepared, genetically modified range of non-foods, with widening girths, increasing rates of diabetes and ever-mounting NHS bills for diseases that could be avoided if only we *all* ate food as nature intended – in its simplest form. We are both proponents of buying British, locally sourced, fresh seasonal produce where possible, and reducing waste by teaching people how to use their food wisely and frugally. We eschew anything that risks being genetically modified, preferring instead to choose an alternative ingredient if we can't be assured that the ones we are using are in their natural state.

We also believe that good food should cost less, but without the knowledge of how to prepare your own from basic ingredients you are forced to pay the market rate for dishes that have been prepared in gigantic kitchens, without love and attention. Food that *is* prepared with love and care *does* taste better – it's an energetic transfer that takes place, and ends up on your tongue, being absorbed in your belly, nourishing the very core of your being. Food is primarily for nourishment, not for punishment or reward, and should be eaten consciously, taking time to be aware of what it affords you and your health. All too often in this frantically busy 21st-century world, we eat while on the hop, or sitting in front of our computers, expecting our digestive systems to 'just take care of it', and not realising that our indigestion, bloated tummies and constipation are a direct result of our unconscious eating. We want to encourage you to take time over your meals, sit around a table with

friends and loved ones, and appreciate the wonderful offering that is the meal on your plate.

So we have written this book together, combining our experience of great cooking with nutritional know-how to inspire you back into your own kitchen, to sample and savour, simmer and sizzle! We want to encourage each and every one of you to try our simple ethos of taking great raw ingredients, in the right combination, cooked to perfection, to nourish your body and soul. Bon appétit!

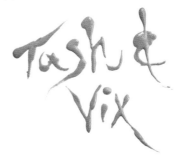

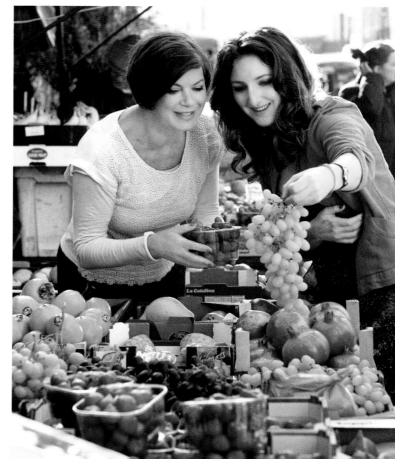

The Foundation of Balanced Eating

What is a balanced way of eating in today's terms? We are constantly bombarded with one diet after another, all of which seek to either negate or contradict the other. We may have heard the benefits of the high-protein, low-carbohydrate approach – guaranteed weight loss, apparently safely – but we already know that cutting out any of the major food groups will leave us wanting, eventually.

What we need, and what we are illustrating in this Honestly Healthy Alkaline Programme, is to have the right balance of *all* three food groups – that is, carbohydrates, proteins and fats (see Know your food groups, page 12), in their cleanest and most natural forms – to suit us individually and ensure that we have all the essential nutrients required for healing and repair, rebuilding and energy production on a day-to-day, moment-to-moment basis.

Benefits of an alkaline approach

How often do you find yourself with indigestion, or burping after a meal? Or, even worse, knowing that you have eaten too much, or too rich or excessively heavy foods? Reaching for coffee or tea to 'help it all go down' is hardly the answer, with alcohol yet another burden on your body's whole digestive system. Yet this is the pattern of the 21st-century Western diet and it is now recognised as a contributing factor to the types of diseases with which we are increasingly faced – diabetes, heart disease and cancers. Many of our frequently chosen foods in the Western diet are acid-forming in the body – that is, when digested they form acidic residues in the bloodstream. Such foods include all meat, dairy produce and processed foods in any form, including sugars, commercial breads, biscuits and cakes. In small amounts this is not harmful, but eating acid-forming foods regularly places a heavier burden on the kidneys and liver to break them down further. Both organs require an increase of certain minerals to 'buffer' such acidity. For example, additional magnesium is required by the kidneys to alkalise waste matter and, if sufficient amounts of this mineral are not available, stores of magnesium may be leached from bone tissue to support kidney function.

Eating predominantly alkaline food is far easier on the whole digestive system, as well as matching the pH of the blood, which runs between 7.35 and 7.45. The Honestly Healthy Alkaline Programme has been designed to provide vegetarian alkaline foods in balanced combinations to guide you through this new way of eating. You will find that, within a few weeks, you will look and feel lighter, your concentration and memory will have sharpened, your energy levels will have soared and the quality of your sleep will have improved dramatically.

Eating alkaline means consuming fresh foods as close to nature as possible – organic wholefoods, predominantly vegetarian, with small amounts of pulses and whole grains to supplement an abundance of fruit and vegetables. These can be raw, lightly cooked or sprouted to create a higher level of protein (see Sprouted beans and seeds, page 34).

Which foods are acid and which are alkaline?

You may be surprised to find that some of the foods you are eating on a daily basis are highly acid-forming (see opposite), contributing to a sense of being over-full, bloated, windy and uncomfortable. Following a primarily alkaline programme will do away with many of these symptoms, virtually overnight. *We are not suggesting that you omit all acidic foods, but rather eat less of them, and ensure that, if you do eat them, you do so alongside plenty of alkaline foods to render the overall meal more alkaline in its total (see also pages 15 and 25).*

Very acid-forming	Mildly acid-forming	Alkaline
STARCHY GRAINS AND VEGETABLES – Breakfast cereals (commercially produced), wheat, gluten-flour breads and pasta, bean (kidney, white), chickpea, peanut butter, pea (dried)	**STARCHY GRAINS AND VEGETABLES** – Buckwheat, corn, lentil, quinoa, millet, oat, rice (white and brown), rye, sweet potato	**STARCHY GRAINS AND VEGETABLES** – Barley, millet, lima bean, soya bean (edamame, fresh or dried), soya lecithin
FATS, OILS AND ESSENTIAL FATS – Cows' dairy produce (including milk, butter, cheese, yogurt, cream and ice cream), ghee	**FATS, OILS AND ESSENTIAL FATS** – Borage oil, Brazil nut, caraway seed, cashew, cumin seed, fennel seed, feta, flax seed, halloumi, hazelnut, linseed oil, macadamia nut, peanut, pumpkin seed, sesame seed and oil, sunflower seed and oil, walnut	**FRUITS** – Apple, apricot, avocado, berry (all), cherry, date, fig, grapefruit, grape, lemon, lime, mango, melon (cantaloupe and watermelon), olives, orange, peach, pear, pineapple, plum, papaya, plums, raisin, rhubarb, sultana, tomato (raw)
PROTEIN – Beef, lamb, mutton, pork, rabbit, chicken, duck, goose, turkey, fish, shellfish, egg, seeds (cooked), gelatine	*NOTE: In this book we include foods that are considered to be strictly acid-forming, such as flax seeds, brown rice or quinoa. We have listed these as 'alkaline' (see page 11, pages 16–19) because their nutrient content is so rich that, when combined with plenty of alkaline-rich foods in the same dish, their content is still predominantly alkaline.*	**NON-STARCHY VEGETABLES** – Alfalfa sprout, artichoke, asparagu, bean (green), beetroot (beet) (including the leaves), broccoli, carrot, cauliflower, celery, chard (all colours), chicory, coconut (fresh water and flesh), dandelion, endive, garlic, greens (winter and summer), horseradish, kale, kelp, kohlrabi, leek, lettuce (all types), mushroom, onion, pea (fresh), pepper, radish, sorrel, spinach, sprouted seed, sprout, squash, turnip, watercress, wheatgrass
		FATS, OILS AND ESSENTIAL FATS – Almonds, coconut oil, olive oil
DRINKS AND CONDIMENTS – All alcohol, coffee, cola drinks, soda water, sugar, tea, tonic water		**DRINKS AND CONDIMENTS** – Almond milk, coconut water (fresh), goat's milk (raw), herbal teas (excepting fruit teas, owing to their tendency to mould spores in the drying process), lemon water, soya milk, water (distilled); agave syrup, apple cider vinegar, cayenne pepper, chilli pepper, cumin (ground), fresh herbs (all), ginger, honey (raw), lemongrass, lime leaves, mustard seeds and paste, sea salt, sea vegetables (including chlorella, kelp, spirulina, wakame), tamari sauce, turmeric

What is alkaline?

There are two sorts of alkaline foods, those that are alkaline to digest in the first place, and those that have an alkaline 'ash' – that is, they become alkaline as a result of being combined with the digestive enzymes produced in the mouth, stomach and small intestine. These are known as alkaline-forming foods, and can often be wrongly observed as 'acidic' to taste – the perfect example of this is lemons and limes, which are acid in taste, but actually very alkalising (see lists of alkalising foods on pages 16–19).

All foods need to be broken down into a form of liquid that can then be absorbed through the intestinal wall into the bloodstream, and it is the minerals that each food contains that dictate primarily whether it is predominantly acidic or alkaline. Generally speaking, those foods higher in potassium, magnesium, calcium, sodium, zinc, copper and iron form a basic ash (that is, in the neutral zone of acid/alkaline, the category into which most natural foods fall).

Simply put, all vegetarian foods such as vegetables and some fruits, nuts, seeds, pulses and whole grains contain a range of predominantly alkaline minerals and are alkalising, while animal produce, along with fermented and caffeinated foods and all processed and fried foods, are acid-forming.

The pH spectrum

The pH spectrum is used to measure the acidity/alkalinity of all sorts of substances – stomach acid is pH 1 while ammonia is pH 14. When it comes to food and drink, pH values centre around pH 3–9. The higher the pH on the scale below, the more alkalising the food.

TESTING YOUR PH LEVELS

Measuring your acid to alkaline ratio can be carried out with litmus testing papers for either urine or saliva, which you can buy from your local pharmacy. Urine is perhaps more accurate, although saliva is quicker and more easily accessible (it can be done over the counter). Ask your pharmacist for either type of testing papers, but note that you cannot test saliva on a urine-test paper – the colour of the litmus will not change.

Urine – The pH of your urine varies according to dehydration and levels of acid-forming foods in the body. Alcohol and caffeine, for instance, substantially change the pH of urine as they are dehydrating and, therefore, make the kidneys work harder to buffer the acidity. Collect a mid-stream sample of urine, dip in the litmus paper strip and wait for the colour change. Compare the colour with the indicators on the container to read off your pH. A healthy urine pH is 6.5–7.25.

Saliva – The pH of your saliva also varies according to what you've eaten or drunk within the last couple of hours. To create enough saliva for testing, activate your tongue in your mouth for 30 seconds and then swallow. Repeat this process twice before placing a litmus paper strip on your tongue ('rinsing' your mouth in this way will ensure a more accurate reading) and then checking the final colour against the indicator on the container to discover your pH. A healthy saliva pH is 6.5–7.5.

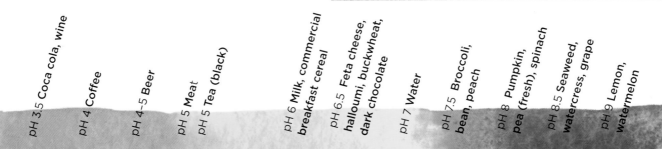

pH 3.5 Coca cola, wine

pH 4 Coffee

pH 4–5 Beer

pH 5 Meat

pH 5 Tea (black)

pH 6 Milk, commercial **breakfast cereal**

pH 6.5 Feta cheese, **halloumi, buckwheat, dark chocolate**

pH 7 Water

pH 7.5 Broccoli, **bean, peach**

pH 8 Pumpkin, **pea (fresh), spinach**

pH 8.5 Seaweed, **watercress, grape**

pH 9 Lemon, **watermelon**

Alkaline foods

Different foods have different levels of alkalising power and we find it useful to divide them into three groups, see below. In the recipe part of the book, we classify each recipe with an alkalising rating so that you can pick and choose meals and snacks to help counterbalance acid-forming foods to achieve a more balanced diet and optimum health.

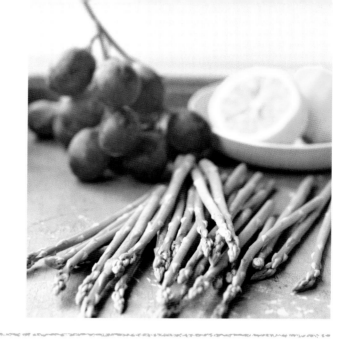

Really Really Alkaline: pH 8.5 to 9

Agar agar, artichoke, asparagus, avocado, broccoli, cauliflower, cayenne pepper, fennel, grapefruit, grape, kale, kelp and seaweed, kiwi fruit, leek, lemon, lime, melon, pineapple, raisin, spinach, tomato (raw), umeboshi plum, vegetable juice (all), watercress

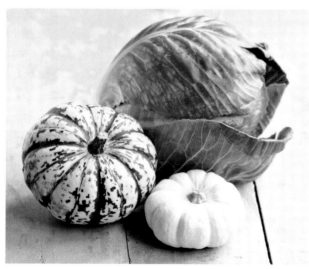

Really Alkaline: pH 7.5 to 8

Alfalfa sprout, apple cider vinegar, apple, apricot, bamboo shoot, banana (firm), bean (green), beetroot (beet), cabbage, carrot, celery, daikon radish, date, fig, guava, kohlrabi, lettuce, mango, nectarine, okra, papaya, parsnip, peach, pear, pea (fresh), pepper, potato, pumpkin, squash, sweetcorn, tamari, turnip

Alkaline: pH 7

Almond, amaranth, aubergine (eggplant), barley malt, berry (all), Brussels sprout, cherry, chestnut, coconut (fresh water and flesh), cucumber, goat's milk (raw), millet, mushroom, olive oil, olive (ripe), onion, pickles, pineapple, radish, sesame seed, soya bean, soya milk, sprouted grains, tempeh, tofu, tomato (cooked), vinegar (other than apple cider vinegar, which is the most alkaline of all vinegars)

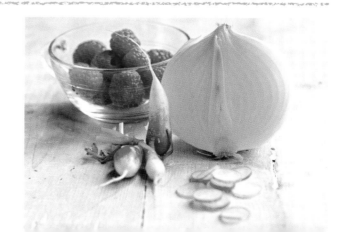

Know Your Food Groups

There always seems to be confusion over what exactly each food contains, and whether or not it can contain more than one compound – is it a carbohydrate, a protein or an essential fat, or might it comprise all three? Here we explain the function of each food group, making the whole subject far easier to understand.

What are the types of carbohydrate?

Carbohydrates are the largest of the three groups, with all fruit and nearly all vegetables, as well as grains, falling within this category. They are the energy providers, being broken down into glucose, which is either used immediately for all physical and mental energy or stored in the muscles and liver as glucose and glycogen until needed. Nourishment is required on a daily basis to stay physically and mentally alert, and if you have ever worked out excessively in a gym, or participated in a marathon, you will know how it feels to literally 'run out of energy' as your muscles can no longer respond to what your mind is asking them to do. This is why marathon runners 'carb-load' in the day or two before the big run. This 'running out of energy' rarely happens on a daily basis, unless you are under-nourishing your body, in which case your body will look to your fat stores for energy. *Feeling ravenous is your body's way of telling you that your glucose stores are running on empty – it's time to pay attention and have a meal before you lose concentration or feel physically exhausted.*

However, the different groups of carbohydrates perform a variety of additional functions, and are digested at different rates.

Grains for essential energy production

All grains (barley, buckwheat, millet, oats, quinoa, rice, rye) contain abundant B vitamins, which are vital for energy production at a cellular level. Each cell in your body (particularly muscle cells) contains tiny powerhouses known as mitochondria, which break down the glucose and convert it into energy. The more you exercise, the more mitochondria you develop per cell, increasing the ability to store and utilize energy. This is one of the reasons that fit people feel good – they are literally walking bundles of energy! Time to get off the sofa and get moving!

Grains also contain a variety of essential minerals required for muscle movement (think beating hearts as well as walking and running), breathing, immune function, metabolism and total body rebuilding and repair. Without grains, the body has to look to its own reserves of fat and lean muscle tissue. Burning fat for fuel is possible, but the energy production in this manner produces a

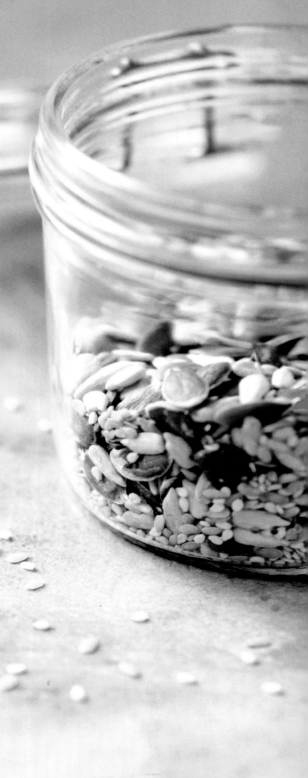

'dirty' fuel, requiring plenty of antioxidant vitamins to 'mop up the mess'. This explains why those who lose a lot of fat quickly often don't feel very well – losing fat gradually and consistently is a far healthier and long-lasting approach. On the other end of the scale, super-fit bodies, such as those of marathon runners, need to consume adequate grains in their diet to ensure that their valuable lean muscle tissue is not broken down at a rate faster than it is rebuilt, otherwise they will lose stamina. Muscle tissue contains the highest number of mitochondria of all tissue in the body.

Mental alertness is dependent on the same type of energy production, and it is a misconception that we can 'do without' the starch and glucose found in grains. It is estimated that the brain actually uses approximately 70% of the energy released from glucose produced through the breaking down of this specific food group in its normal everyday function (carbohydrates are the main glucose-producing foods). If sitting in a lecture, concentrating on driving or giving a talk or demonstration, the energy requirements can rise to 85–90% of all the glucose stored, which explains why speakers such as politicians and lecturers often eat immediately after their speech is delivered – they have exhausted their stored energy. You may find that in order to focus on reading this part of the book, you need a quick-fix snack to stay focused – grabbing a banana or a couple of oatcakes will do the trick.

Many 'slimming diets' of late have propounded a low- or no-starch at all approach, meaning that once the fat stores are depleted, the body must turn to breaking down lean muscle tissue for energy. Think of the images you have witnessed of emaciated or anorexic bodies gracing the popular magazines in today's world – these may be thin bodies, but they are not healthy ones! We *need* carbohydrates! This is why many of the recipes in this book contain grains, either in salads, breads or soups – remember that they are the energy part of the meal.

Simple or complex – that is the question

Whether it be in its wholegrain form (think oats or millet for porridge (oatmeal), brown or red Camargue rice for risotto or whole quinoa for savory or sweet dishes), or ground into flours for wholegrain pasta, breads and crackers, these are the complex form of the grain – unaltered and unadulterated. They have the very goodness of the grain left intact, including the fibre, vitamins and minerals, and have been used for several thousand years as the very staff of life.

Simple carbohydrates, on the other hand, are those that have been bleached, blanched, milled several times to form white flour, white rice, white bread, and all the produce that such processing brings. Commercial cereals, for instance, literally melt on your tongue (as there is no real fibre or goodness left in them!), and mass-produced biscuits and cakes require abundant sugars, sweeteners and other additives to help make them taste of anything. The goodness has literally been wrung out of them, and they have nothing to offer in the way of nutrition. This is why those who start a pack of biscuits can rarely stop before the pack is finished, as their body searches for something to convert into energy – contrast this to eating a couple of slices of filling and nourishing pumpernickel bread, and you instantly realise why choosing the complex variety is the only way to go!

Fruits and vegetables for instant energy

Also falling under the carbohydrate banner are fruits and vegetables, providing energy at a more rapidly available rate – think of how quickly you gain momentum after eating a banana or apple at virtually any time of the day. *Fruit that is eaten on an empty stomach is digested in under 20 minutes, with the sugars inherently found in such fruits providing instant glucose for energy.*

Root vegetables, those that grow under the ground (think carrots, white and sweet potatoes, turnips, parsnips, etc), all contain abundant glucose stores, as they derive their goodness and nutrients directly from the moisture in the soil surrounding them. So too those vegetables that grow sitting on the earth (think butternut squash, pumpkin and courgettes (zucchini)), while these also derive energy directly from the sun. They are packed with antioxidant vitamins and minerals, and should form a large part of our daily eating. We include all of these energy-packed ground vegetables in the Honestly Healthy recipes, as we know that the natural sweetness they provide, together with their vitalising minerals, will satisfy everyone's palate – whether spiced or natural, these foods are essential to the Honestly Healthy Alkaline Programme.

Green vegetables, which grow above ground, have the added benefits of chlorophyll, the deep green colour derived from the energy from sunlight that is the 'blood' of the plant. Chlorophyll is one of the most alkalising compounds provided in our food, and should be included, in some form, at least twice a day, in as natural a state as possible.

At Honestly Healthy, we believe that these life-enhancing foods should form the major part of your daily meals – alkaline in their natural state, and packed with energy (see also Stacking foods, page 22). *The variety of colour and texture in above- or below-ground-growing vegetables is key to providing your body with the widest range of cell-protecting antioxidants, energy-producing glucose and immune-enhancing minerals.*

What are the types of protein?

While all natural food is life-giving, it is the proteins that are *life-building*. All proteins are broken down into amino acids, known as the *building blocks* of life. All animal produce contains the eight essential amino acids we require to rebuild and repair. However, they can be acid-forming in the body, taking days to digest and often putrefying on the way through the digestive system, forming waste products that can be toxic and exhausting, as well as causing bloating and indigestion.

Conversely, vegetarian proteins are found in any food that can be planted to grow into a grain, plant or tree – in other words, often many, many times the size of the original seed. Think transformation of the sunflower seed into the 2.5–3m (8–10ft) flower – gigantic, given the original size of the seed. These foods are far simpler to digest, and yet yield the same building blocks for every cell in our bodies. It is vital, however, to combine the different sources of vegetarian proteins in order to acquire all eight essential amino acids that together make up our bodies. The perfect analogy for this 'building' process is to think of a collection of Lego bricks and the myriad shapes and objects that can be built with their different pieces, colours and shapes.

THE TRIAD OF PROTEINS

Grains, legumes and pulses are important because they provide different types of amino acids, coming together to create total proteins. Legumes include all the beans – butter beans, chickpeas, black-eyed beans, kidney beans – all of which are included in abundance in our recipes. Pulses such as lentils, split peas and dhal are the third group that make up this essential triad of proteins.

All nuts and seeds are perfect protein sources. In your childhood classroom you would have marvelled at the broad-bean-in-the-jar session in Elementary Biology – where the two cotyledons (two halves of the bean) split open to allow both the root and the shoot to appear. All beans, nuts and seeds (as well as most grains) can be sprouted in this way and, as *living food* (literally still growing!), these choices of proteins are the most life-giving, body-building you can have. Including some in your salads on a regular basis will reap numerous benefits – both visible and internal. Nuts and seeds are also vital providers of the essential fatty acids that make up the largest portion of our brains and nervous system (see Fats opposite).

Soya-based produce is one of the only complete proteins available for the vegetarian, alkaline way. Soya beans (choose non-GM sources) contain all eight amino acids and, in their natural state, preserve them for full use in the body. However, in broken-down form, such as soy sauce, tofu and tempeh, this complete protein source is actually disrupted, so it is wise to ensure a regular intake of the edamame bean (Japanese for soya bean). The only other complete protein from a vegetarian source is blue–green algae, spirulina and chlorella (see also pages 34–35).

What are the types of fat?

Fats – always a source of anxiety to those who don't understand that some fat is not only good for you, but *essential* – come in various forms.

Fats that are good for you

The simplest way to explain those fats that are good for you is to think of the life-*building* proteins, such as nuts and seeds, and realise that these are usually coupled with (and work in conjunction with) the essential fats found within them. So, sunflower and pumpkin seed oils, macadamia and coconut oils, together with walnut, hazelnut and olive oils are all beneficial fats, supporting nerve function, mental alertness, concentration and memory. **Indeed, some 75% of the brain itself is made up of essential fats.** Were you to hold a brain in your hands, you would be amazed at how 'fatty' an organ it is. Packed with nerves, this brilliant computer in your body is protected and carried within a massive amount of essential fatty acid tissue – miraculous.

In the same way, the insulation of our bodies – the protective layer called our skin – is made up of trillions of cells formed from what is known as a phospholipid bi-layer. This is a double layer of essential fats around every cell. It is easy to spot someone on a low-fat/no-fat diet, as their skin is wrinkled and dried, and literally starved of essential fatty acids – just think what their inner organs look like if their outer skin is so parched. Our skin not only insulates us from the heat and cold of our environment, but also envelops our bodies in a protective layer. As the skin is the largest organ of elimination in the body, it is vital to keep its outer layer hydrated with essential fats ingested from within to allow the toxins out. Dehydrated skin lacks not only water but also essential fats to keep each cell supple.

Fats that are bad for you

Saturated fats are found in animal fats – think bacon, sausages, lamb fat, goose fat, cheeses and so forth. These fats become damaged in the presence of heat, light and air, and especially in cooking. Research has illustrated that cooked red meat eaten on a regular basis has a role to play in colon cancer – perhaps because it sits partially undigested in the gut for days, but also because of these damaging fats. These fats clog up the arteries, causing heart disease and stroke.

Reversing the damage

Interestingly, the benefits of the essential fats found in nuts and seeds and their oils can *undo* the damage the bad fats have caused. This is because the essential fatty acids, known as omega-3, -6, -9 and -12, are predominantly anti-inflammatory, whereas saturated fats have been found to be pro-inflammatory. Many life-threatening diseases are caused in part by inflammation (see also page 22).

We at Honestly Healthy ensure that we look to choosing several forms of these beneficial essential fats every day. We infuse bottles of olive, coconut, sunflower and hemp oils with herbs, spices and garlic to create complex flavours for salads and vegetables.

A little word about fish

Much is known about the rich sources of omega-3 essential fats found in oily fish, such as tuna, herring, mackerel and salmon. However, to maximise the fish's full nutritional value, we suggest you buy wild varieties wherever possible and avoid intensively farmed fish.

Alkalinity rating	Nutrients	Benefits to the body
Vegetables		
♥♥♥ Artichoke	Calcium, magnesium, potassium, sodium, folic acid, beta-carotene and vitamins C and K	Diuretic, digestive, contains inulin (stimulates good bacteria in the gut), supports liver and promotes bile flow
♥♥♥ Asparagus	Potassium, folic acid, vitamins C and K and beta-carotene	Kidney-stimulating, mildly laxative and antibacterial
♥♥♥ Broccoli	Calcium, magnesium, phosphorus, vitamins B3, B5 and C and folic acid	Antioxidant, intestinal cleanser, antiviral, antibiotic and stimulates liver function
♥♥♥ Cauliflower	Calcium, magnesium, folic acid, potassium, boron, beta-carotene and vitamin C	Excellent antioxidant, supports liver and kidney disorders and relieves high blood pressure and constipation
♥♥♥ Fennel	Calcium, magnesium, sodium, potassium, vitamin C, folic acid and phytoestrogens	Antispasmodic, relieves cramps, helps to digest fats and good for weight control
♥♥♥ Kale	Calcium, magnesium, phosphorus, potassium, vitamins C, E and K, folic acid and iodine	Supports thyroid and metabolism, detoxes stomach, improves digestion, stimulates immune system, kills errant bacteria and viruses, and is a potent antioxidant
♥♥♥ Kelp	Iodine, calcium, iron and potassium	Highest source of these minerals, benefits cardiovascular and nervous systems, cleanses toxins and aids digestion
♥♥♥ Leek	Calcium, potassium, folic acid and vitamins A and K	Cleansing, diuretic and eliminates uric acid in gout
♥♥♥ Spinach	Iron, calcium, magnesium, folic acid and vitamins B6 and C	Helps regulate blood pressure, anti-cancer properties, boosts immunity and supports bone health
♥♥♥ Tomato, raw	Calcium, magnesium, phosphorus, folic acid, beta-carotene and vitamin C	Antiseptic, antibacterial, supports liver function and reduces inflammation
♥♥♥ Watercress	Calcium, magnesium, phosphorus, vitamin C, beta-carotene, iron and iodine	Diuretic, breaks up kidney or bladder stones, purifies blood, reduces mucus in digestive and nasal tracts and helps increase metabolism

Alkalinity rating	Nutrients	Benefits to the body
♥♥ Beetroot (Beet)	Calcium, magnesium potassium, vitamin C and manganese	Cleansing, reduces kidney stones and detoxes liver and gall bladder
♥♥ Carrot	Calcium, magnesium, potassium and beta-carotene	Cleanses liver, encourages detoxing and supports eye function
♥♥ Celery	Calcium, magnesium, sodium, folic acid and vitamin B3	Helps lower blood pressure, aids digestion, prevents fermentation in the gut and helps prevent arthritis
♥♥ Garlic	Calcium, phosphorus, vitamin C and potassium	Potent antispasmodic, antibacterial and lowers cholesterol
♥♥ Ginger	Calcium, magnesium, potassium and phosphorus	Antispasmodic, anti-nausea, stimulates liver and gall bladder and improves circulation,
♥ Onion	Calcium, magnesium, potassium, folic acid, phosphorus and quercetin	Anti-inflammatory, antiseptic, antibiotic, reduces spasms in asthmatics, removes heavy metals and parasites, and is a potent cleanser of digestive tract
♥ Tomato, cooked	Calcium, magnesium, phosphorus, folic acid, beta-carotene and vitamin C	Antiseptic, antibacterial, supports liver function and reduces inflammation

Fruits

Alkalinity rating	Nutrients	Benefits to the body
♥♥♥ Avocado	Potassium, folic acid and vitamins B3, B5, E and K	High-protein fruit, calming, good for digestion and prevents anaemia
♥♥♥ Grapefruit	Calcium, magnesium, vitamin C and potassium	Relieves arthritic pain through salicylic acid, blood cleansing, supports heart health and prevents calcium deposits
♥♥♥ Lemon/lime	Potassium and vitamin C	Dissolves gallstones, potent antiseptic and natural antibiotic
♥♥ Apple	Potassium, vitamin C, beta-carotene and pectin	A tonic, cleansing, lowers cholesterol and removes toxins
♥♥ Date	Calcium, iron, vitamin B3 and beta-carotene	Relieves diarrhoea and supports respiratory system

Alkalinity rating	Nutrients	Benefits to the body
♥♥ Fig	Calcium, potassium, vitamin C and beta-carotene	Mild laxative, clears toxins and high source of calcium
♥♥ Mango	Vitamin C, beta-carotene, potassium, calcium and magnesium	Reduces acidity, supports kidneys, relieves poor digestion and is a good blood cleanser
♥♥ Papaya	Calcium, magnesium, potassium, vitamin C and beta-carotene	Potent antioxidant, anti-parasitic, soothes intestinal inflammation, reduces wind and is a good cleanser
♥♥ Pear	Calcium, magnesium, potassium, folic acid, iodine and pectin	Diuretic, benefits thyroid, stimulates metabolism and pectin removes toxins from gut
♥ Coconut	Magnesium, zinc, potassium, folic acid and vitamin C	Very rehydrating and helps to regulate/support thyroid metabolism in energy production
♥ Pineapple	Calcium, magnesium, potassium, beta-carotene and vitamin C	Antispasmodic, contains bromelain (good for digestion) and clears bacteria and parasites

Grains and Pulses

Alkalinity rating	Nutrients	Benefits to the body
♥ Barley (see page 25)	Potassium, zinc, magnesium, calcium, B vitamins and folic acid	Soothes digestion and supports liver function, heals stomach ulcers and lowers cholesterol
♥ Brown rice (see page 25)	Calcium, magnesium, iron, potassium, zinc, vitamins B3, B5 and B6 and folic acid	Calming, mood-enhancing and energising
♥ Buckwheat (see page 25)	Calcium, magnesium, zinc, potassium, beta-carotene, vitamin C, essential fatty acids and rutin	Grain with complete protein content and supports cardiovascular system and micro-circulation
♥ Chickpea (see page 25)	Calcium, magnesium, potassium, zinc, beta-carotene, folic acid, phosphorus and manganese	Supports kidneys and is a digestive cleanser
♥ Lentil (see page 25)	Calcium, magnesium, potassium, zinc and folic acid	Good source of alkaline minerals for every organ of the body and neutralises lactic acid produced in muscles during exercise

Alkalinity rating	Nutrients	Benefits to the body
♥ Quinoa (see page 25)	Calcium, magnesium, potassium and vitamin B3	Gluten-free, high-protein and high-calcium grain with antiviral properties
♥ Soya bean	Calcium, potassium, magnesium and vitamins A, C, K and B3	Complete vegetarian protein, lowers cholesterol and balances hormones

Nuts and Seeds

Alkalinity rating	Nutrients	Benefits to the body
♥ Almond	Calcium, magnesium, potassium, zinc, folic acid and vitamins B and E	Good protein source, calming, sedating and a skin food
♥ Macadamia nut (see page 25)	Calcium, potassium, low sodium, high fibre and high in essential fats (monounsaturated)	Removes toxins, lowers cholesterol and contains anti-aging oils
♥ Sunflower seed (see page 25)	Calcium, magnesium, vitamins A, B-complex, D, E and K, zinc, manganese and omega-3 and -6 essential fats	Perfect little buds of protein – more so than eggs, meat or dairy; supports eye health and pectin removes toxins and heavy metals from the gut
♥ Walnut (see page 25)	Potassium, calcium, magnesium, zinc, folic acid, vitamins C and E and omega-3 and -6 essential fats	Supports kidney and lung function, potent source of essential fats for brain, cognitive function and mood regulation and improves metabolism

Miscellaneous

Alkalinity rating	Nutrients	Benefits to the body
♥♥ Coconut water	Magnesium, zinc, potassium, folic acid and vitamin C	Very rehydrating, helps to regulate/ support thyroid metabolism in energy production
♥ Tofu	Calcium, magnesium potassium, iron and vitamins A and K	Perfect source of protein for vegetarians, lowers cholesterol and balances hormones

Learn New Eating Habits

When it comes to taking a new approach to healthy eating, it's not just what you eat that matters, it's also the way in which you eat. Do you find you're always grabbing food on the run? Or don't eat for ages and then end up eating too much? So, now is the time for making positive change in both how much and the way you eat so that they become the norm for you.

Choosing the right portion size

There are many ideas around portion sizes, the most prevalent being to measure your portions on scales, or by their fat or calorie content. We don't believe that is either healthy or balanced, and can't imagine how thousands of people are bound by these archaic methods that now bear no relevance to our everyday living. The old ethos of calories in/calories out is over-simplistic, and binds you to your bathroom scales, your tape measures and your kitchen weights. The only reason we give such detailed measurements in our recipe section is to guide you when you start – we then actively encourage you to experiment according to your own taste – a pinch of this, a spoon of that.

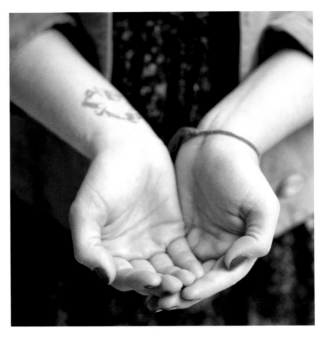

Hand cupping – *your* hands for *your* stomach

In nutritional terms, we recommend opting for a more manual way of controlling your portion sizes so that you are no longer 'bound' to measurements that are so limiting. In the photo (on the right), we have shown you the most straightforward way to measure the amount of food that is right for *you* – cup your hands together, and *your* hands will guide *you* to the correct amount for *your* stomach – for it is now known that *the size of one of your hands roughly equates to the size of your stomach (each of us has a stomach shape and size as individual as a fingerprint)*.

While this might look small, if you were to pile your entire meal into your cupped hands and then spread it on a plate, you would then see that it is more than enough – it is simply that we are used to being served so much more than this in the typical Western diet.

Remember, we are not dieting here – we are creating principles that we can adhere to for life, and trust that it works for each of us, without going into the endless mind conversations – 'I shouldn't have that...' or 'that was too much...' – that plague too many, mindlessly. To set standard measurements is irrelevant when each of us is so individual – how can a 6'4" man be expected to eat as little as a 5'2" petite woman? Hence *your* hands for *your* stomach.

It is something of a myth that eating excessively stretches the stomach, or that starving does the opposite – if you haven't eaten for a couple of days,

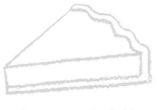
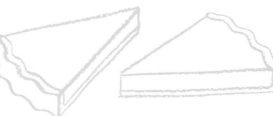
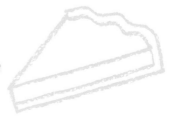

and then do so, your stomach is bound to groan a little. Rather, when you are used to overeating, you probably don't know when you are full as you are likely to be eating 'mindlessly' (see Eating conciously, below).

Smaller bowls and plates

We recommend that you build a collection of smaller bowls and plates than you usually use. The fashion has been to serve meals on the largest plates possible, as this resembles restaurant eating, but what one forgets is that restaurants usually serve small portions on large plates to make them look more dramatic! Be honest with yourself and clear out and reorganise your cupboards. Use the extra-large dinner plates as serving plates, and finger bowls as soup bowls for starters. If you are having a one-pot meal (such as Butternut Squash Risotto, page 129), then choose a regular size soup bowl (18cm/7in bowl area with extra for rim) or a small, deep serving bowl (12–15cm/5–6in diameter) as this is the only dish you will be eating from. A 25cm/10in dinner plate is ample for all the recipes and combination of dishes that we have suggested in our recipe section – and these need not be filled to the edge (see Stacking foods, page 22).

Eating consciously

How often are you aware of what you are eating? Do you stop to savour the look, texture and colour of your food, or do you shovel your meal in as quickly as possible? All too often, we eat on the run, in a furious attempt to 'grab and go'. Yet this is the worst way we can put food and nourishment into our bodies, as we are doing so in a mindless way – it is no wonder, then, that we aren't aware when we are full. Many people eat far too quickly and don't know when they have had enough. Our bodies are designed with a wonderful mechanism called the vagus nerve, which connects the stomach to the hippocampus, the part of the brain that deals with satiety. ***When we eat rapidly, and without concentration, the messages the brain sends via this nerve to the stomach to let us know that we have had enough go largely unnoticed.*** Little wonder that we have a society full of seriously overweight people, as we eat sitting in front of the television, our computers and phones. We are simply not *aware*.

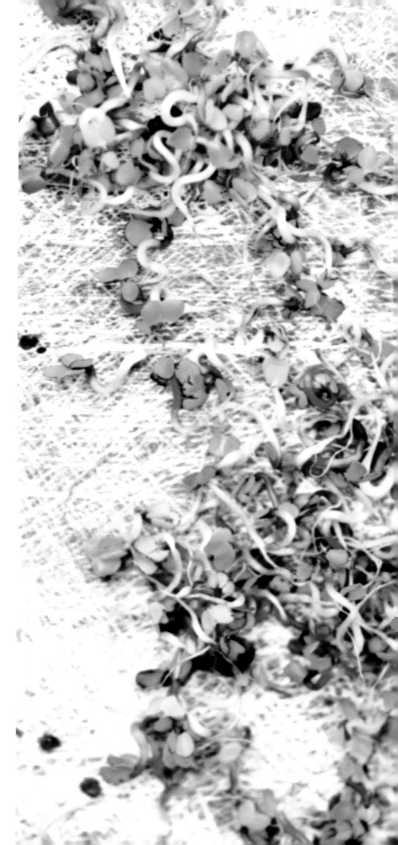

The ABC of conscious eating

A – Allocate time to eat, unfettered, and predominantly as an activity in its own right. Aim to set aside at least 20 minutes for a main meal, and preferably considerably more, without engaging in anything other than conversation with others at the table – banish books, newspapers, television, radio and iPods, and contemplate exactly *what is on your plate*.

B – Be engaged – notice the colour, texture and type of foods in front of you. A meal isn't simply meat, vegetables and potatoes any more (in this case, there is no meat at all, but plenty of building proteins derived from vegetarian sources, such as nuts, grains, sprouted seeds, soya products and some cheeses).

C – Chew your foods thoroughly, putting down your knife and fork between each mouthful, rather than shovelling in the next before you have even finished the first. Take sufficient time to ensure that the enzymes in your mouth (secreted by the parotid glands in the base of the mouth, and mixed with saliva) can mix with your food to break it down into almost a liquid. Try this the next time you eat, and ask yourself, 'Do I munch, munch, swallow... – or do I chew to a juice?' Many yogic practices dictate chewing each mouthful 30–50 times prior to swallowing, to ensure proper digestion. While this is perhaps not practical on a day-to-day basis, the fundamentals of the teaching are sound. No one chokes on liquids, but many do on chunks of food when eating in haste! *This ancient practice of eating mindfully and slowly actually renders a completely different taste to your foods, as chewing and mixing food with enzymes in the saliva renders the food far sweeter than its original components.* This is particularly good for those who feel they are lacking sugary or sweet foods when they start the Honestly Healthy Alkaline Programme.

Stacking foods

The important thing in this method is to know how your portions should be split up into the correct balance of carbohydrates, proteins and essential fats, all of which should be included in each main meal (see right). By including all these food groups in your meal by stacking your foods, you'll eat a healthy and balanced meal each and every time. (See also Know your food groups, page 12.)

Building your stack
With our Stacking method, all these questions become far simpler – think of building a house from the foundations up, see illustration opposite, though it's not possible to show the top layer.

Coconut shavings, the nut and seed butters and oils, the olive oil and lemon dressings are the coating, providing essential fats for our nervous systems and the suppleness of our inner and outer layers of skin. **10%–15% total of dish**

Nuts, seeds, sprouts, tofu, tempeh, beans and pulses are the sprinkling third layer of the dish, which provide the very building and repair blocks of our food. These generally take longer to chew, longer to digest and slow down the release of energy from the dish as a whole. **20%–25% total of dish**

Roasted, grilled, baked, steamed or raw vegetables form the next layer of the stack, providing fibre, vitamins and minerals that mainly alkalise the whole dish, creating colour and contrast (vital not only for the appearance, but also the texture and variety of nutrients contained in the dish). **30%–35% total of dish**

Grains or potatoes always form the bottom of the stack, for example, quinoa, millet, oats, rye, rice or buckwheat. (These complex carbohydrates produce long-lasting energy, providing the very foundation of the stack and the bulk of the dish). **30%–35% total of dish**

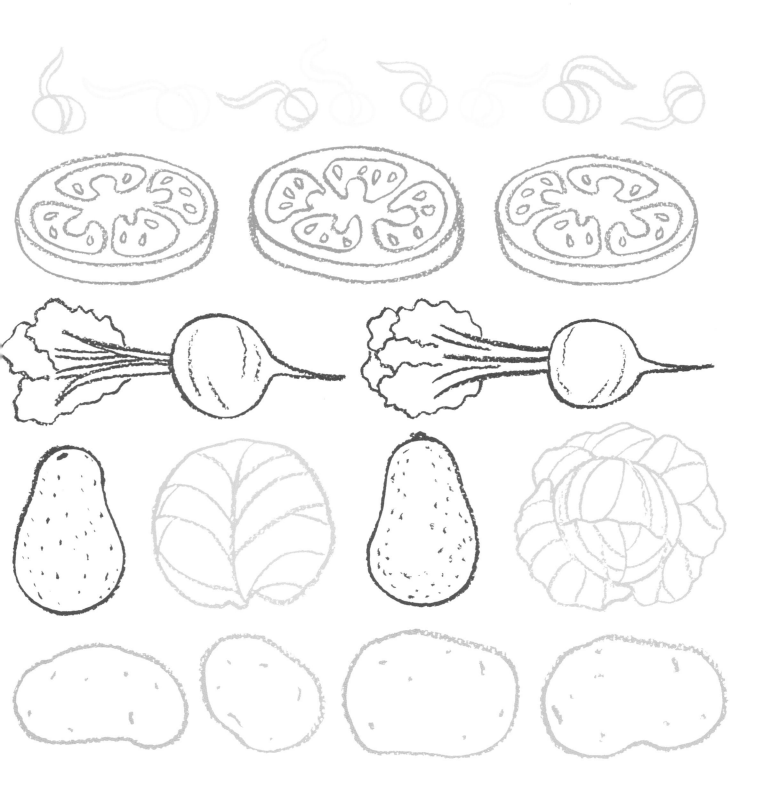

Prevention Before Cure

All too often, we wait until illness occurs before changing our eating and lifestyle habits. At Honestly Healthy, we know how *well* you can feel if you take care of yourself and make sure that illness rarely happens. This is a choice and, while it takes time and dedication, the rewards of ongoing good health are so abundant that we want to encourage you to start aiming for great health, rather than simply good health.

How a 'dis-ease' is created in the body

Our immunity is vital to our overall health, with an army of different types of immune cells present in our bloodstream, but especially in the digestive tract, as this is our interface with the outside world. *It is estimated that as much as 70% of the total of our immune cells are present in the gut –* which we experience in a major way when we have an upset tummy or, worse, food poisoning. These immune cells are present throughout the length of our digestive tract from our mouth to our bowels, ensuring that any pathogenic invaders are quelled at the appropriate point or expedited through the system as fast as possible.

Recognising your body's toxicity

Take a good look at the toxic symptoms in the box (right) and discover how burdened your body's system actually is.

Toxic symptoms

You may be surprised to recognise just how many of these symptoms apply to you:

Headaches/migraines
Joint and/or muscle pain
Indigestion
Heartburn
Bloating
Constipation
Diarrhoea
Stomach cramps
Bad breath
Metallic taste in mouth
Sensitive gums
Food intolerances
Excessively painful menstruation

Watery or itchy eyes
Shortness of breath
Sweating
Skin irritations (eczema, psoriasis)
Dry skin
Unexplained hair loss
Lank or dull hair
Acne or constantly spotty skin
Cellulite
Insomnia
Broken sleep
Fatigue

Mood swings
Depression
Lack of motivation
Inability to focus on anything
Irritability
Anger
Sugar cravings
Salty food cravings
Food bingeing

Some of these symptoms can be due to other causes, but by following the Honestly Healthy Alkaline Programme for just three weeks, you will find that many of these symptoms simply disappear. Why not make the investment of this time and see for yourself?

Allergies and intolerances may be the key

Food allergies are those reactions that are immediate, severe and potentially life-threatening, such as swelling of the mouth and lips and closing of the back of the throat, preventing air getting to the lungs. This is called anaphylaxis, and fortunately occurs relatively rarely. However, food intolerances occur far more frequently, sometimes being more difficult to detect as the reaction can occur up to 70 hours or so after the offending food has been eaten. There are several different ways of testing food sensitivities and, generally speaking, blood tests provide by far the most reliable results, as it is in the bloodstream that most reactions occur.

On a more practical level, keeping a detailed 'food and symptom' diary may well provide you with some simple answers without having to wait for blood tests to be taken. For example, *if you are suffering from severe headaches on a regular basis, plot a chart over the course of a few weeks of when they occur and see how frequently the foods that you eat almost daily tie in with those.*

Well-recognised links to headaches include chocolate (commercially produced, including sugars and sweeteners rather than the more natural cacao and agave, yacon and xylitol alternatives included in our recipes); cheese, red wine and caffeine, all of which contain compounds that are linked with migraines and severe headaches.

Hives and other skin rashes are often associated with strawberries and other red fruits (which can be overly acidic to the body, despite being sweet to taste). Lesser-known links include wheat-based products such as bread, biscuits and cakes with fatigue and mild depression, eggs with joint and muscle aches and pains, and mushrooms, yeast and moulds with chronic fatigue, perpetual flu-like symptoms and low energy and mood.

What is going on here?

The answer is *inflammation*
Inflammation is now considered to be the major cause of most chronic diseases, including heart and cardiovascular, lung and digestive problems, skin problems. Inflammation of *any* tissue in the body attracts extra fluid to the site, and an imbalance of electrolytes (such as sodium, potassium, calcium and magnesium) at a cellular level is commonly found as a result of such inflammation. It is precisely this electrolyte balance that the body is seeking to maintain on a moment-to-moment basis.

Top foods for alkaline energy

We list our top foods, which are included in most of our recipes, with their alkalinity ratings and what they do for your body on the tables on pages 16–19. We always aim to create menu plans that are high in variety and balanced in acid/alkaline content, looking for the magic 80:20 rule – aiming to eat approximately 80% alkaline foods with each meal, or during each day, will go a long way towards ensuring that you are supporting your body's natural functions. We don't have to keep repeating it – you just have to try it!

Magic minerals
The minerals calcium, magnesium, potassium and phosphorus are found in all alkaline foods, and these are the vital minerals for regulating the pH of the body's fluids. Calcium and magnesium also work in balance to regulate the beat of the heart, the building of bone and ligaments, the regulation and response of the nervous system, cognitive function and mood. Both iron and iodine are required for blood transport, for cardiovascular health and for metabolism, which is regulated by the thyroid gland.

Perfect proteins
It is important to note that protein is found in any nut, seed or grain that can be planted and will grow into a tree or flower that is substantially larger than the seed – remember that sunflower, which is many thousands of times larger than the seed it originated from. Soya beans and tofu provide all eight essential amino acids for rebuilding and repair, strong immunity and energy production.

In some recipes in the book, you will see that we have included foods that are considered to be acid-forming, such as brown rice, quinoa, lentils or macadamia nuts. We have listed these as 'alkaline' in the tables on pages 16–19 and include them because their nutrient content is so rich that, when placed with plenty of alkaline-rich foods in the same dish, the combined, or average, alkaline content is still predominantly alkaline. Nature would never have supplied us with these foods had they not had their own benefits. This is a perfect example of when to allow some of the acid-forming foods into your programme – we use some non-cows' dairy produce, such as feta and halloumi, as these are less acid-forming than cows' dairy and provide essential calcium and minerals – but always serve these alongside really really alkaline vegetables, dressings or salads. Remember, the more natural the state of the food, the higher the alkaline content.

How an alkaline state can help to cure ailments

Eating a highly acid-forming, animal-protein-based diet may lead to intestinal inflammation (ulcerative colitis, irritable bowel syndrome (IBS) and Crohn's disease all being at the worst end of the spectrum), as well as chronic rhinitis and skin problems (such as eczema and psoriasis). As meat is difficult to digest, and dairy- and wheat-based foods are commonly eaten daily, it is no wonder that so many people are plagued by a collection of minor illnesses. Sadly, few doctors understand – or even know of – the connection between the foods we choose to eat and the illnesses that occur as a result.

The good news is that once we know how to balance acid and alkaline foods in our diet, massive change can take place. Within a matter of days of removing foods that are causing either inflammation or intolerances, aches and pains start to disappear as the body starts to heal and repair. This is why we recommend the Cleanse phase (see pages 32–37), whereby *all* the potentially offending foods and drinks are removed, toxins are reduced in the environment around you and an abundance of life-giving, energetic foods (such as hemp seed, chlorella and spirulina) are recommended to cleanse the body and alkalise the system; and subsequently the Lifestyle phase (see pages 38–42), which is a programme for life, to ensure increasingly good health.

Alkalising foods begin by literally 'balancing' each cell in the body, supporting its natural energy production and waste-clearing processes by creating the correct electrolyte balance of sodium and potassium. Without getting too technical, the vitality of a cell depends upon sufficient nutrients to allow it to function at its best, and this happens far more readily in an alkaline environment. If the fluids surrounding each cell are too acidic, the sodium/potassium balance is thrown into disarray, causing cellular dehydration. When we talk about 'hydrating' the body, we don't just mean 'drink plenty of water' – we are talking about nutrient-rich juices, green smoothies and alkalising pH drops to add to your water. These are now readily available in most health food shops and online worldwide (see Directory of food suppliers, page 192).

Take the test and see!

We recommend that you drink at least two juices daily over a period of ten days to evaluate improvements to whatever is troubling you at present – headaches, recurrent colds and infections, aches and pains. As your body starts to rebalance its pH levels, your symptoms will start to diminish and the power of eating the alkaline way will be revealed.

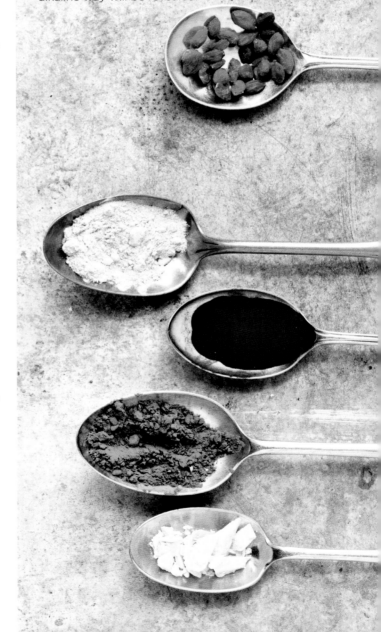

What's Your Fix?

It is inevitable that there are some foods you will find hard to give up – it is little wonder, as they were designed to be addictive in the first place! If you think of the cocktail of sugars and sweeteners, additives and salt included in commercial cereals or breads, for example, the flour and the water used to bring them together are almost incidental when you read the ingredients list!

However, it *is* important to look carefully at just how much of these types of foods you consume on a daily basis, and this is especially relevant when looking at the acid/alkaline balance, for most of these ingredients are acid-forming – and the irony is that it is partly the fact that they *are* acid-forming that makes them so addictive. **By embarking on a predominantly alkaline eating programme, you will find yourself less drawn to them in the first place, and they will eventually become totally unappealing as your palate changes.**

Food addictions and cravings are usually indicative of a body out of balance and signify specific nutrient deficiencies. While most vitamins are readily available in all fruits and vegetables, it is the minerals in whole grains, nuts and seeds, as well as soya products, that nourish us at a cellular level, leaving us feeling satisfied, calm and yet energised. Getting off the junk-food gravy train is key to feeling fantastic, and it deserves the time and effort it initially takes to wean yourself off such foods in order to gain the benefits.

Acknowledging your triggers

Most of us have specific situations that trigger eating 'quick-fix' foods with no real value to us, and it is important to identify them so you can be prepared for the eventuality and provide better choices.

Ask yourself which negative emotions (such as being bored, tired or premenstrual) or particular situations (such as working late or skipping breakfast) are most likely to cause you to pick up a packet of biscuits, crisps, bar of chocolate or salted nuts, alcohol or fizzy drinks, or yet another coffee. It may be that you experience such emotions

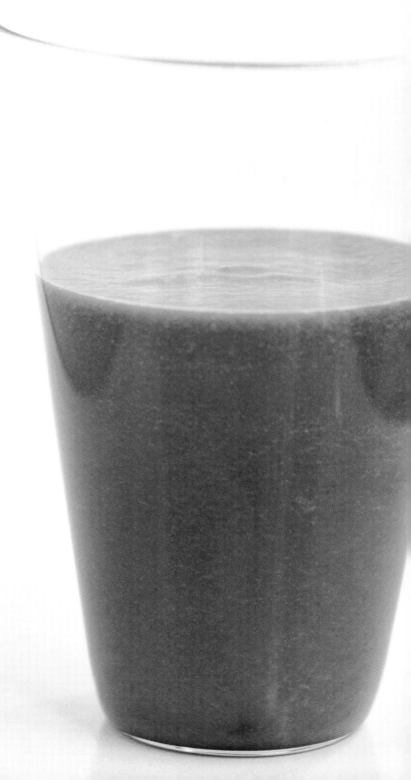

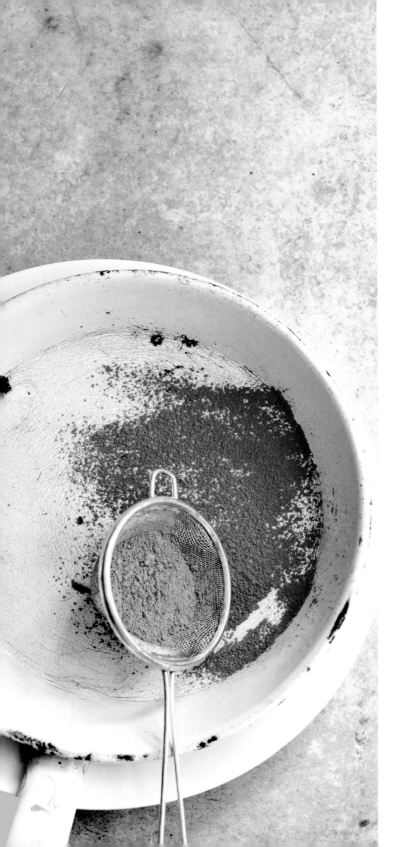

or situations on a regular basis, and frequently give yourself excuses for 'needing' or 'deserving' a treat. But are these foods and drinks really treats, and do they make you feel better at all?

The important thing to remember is that any foods or drinks that give you an instant boost are likely to leave you feeling lower subsequently than before you ate or drank them. This is because any additives, sugars and sweeteners, caffeinated drinks and other stimulants interfere with the delicate balance of your blood-sugar regulation. This leaves you on a perpetual roller coaster of highs and lows, always ending on a low – more tired, more irritable and less motivated to take care of yourself properly.

Start your day as you mean to go on

We recommend that you start your day with a tonic of alkaline goodness. There is nothing more effective than a green smoothie or juice in the morning for regulating blood-sugar levels from the outset (see pages 24 and 46–48). Adding a small amount of protein to your juice, such as ground hemp seed or flax seed, will prolong the release of energy that you derive from such a drink, and prevent the peaks and troughs associated with strong coffee or tea. How you start your day determines how the rest of the day will work for you, as choosing croissants or toast and marmalade will have you reaching for more of the same for the next few hours, eventually leading to fatigue and inability to concentrate. It only takes a few minutes to prepare a fresh juice and ours are designed to be a whole meal in themselves.

Having your cake and eating it too

Looking through our Breads section (see pages 160–163), you will realise that good-quality, wholegrain breads, made without sugar and using sweeteners such as cinnamon, nutmeg, coconut and agave syrup, allow you to indulge in delicious alternatives, rich in B vitamins for energy and minerals that support the immune, nervous and cardiovascular systems. Where these recipes also include nuts and seeds, the protein will provide you with longer-lasting energy, and cooking them at a low temperature preserves the essential fatty acids inherent in all nuts and seeds.

Banishing the chocoholic blues

Cacao, the raw ingredient used to make all chocolate, actually contains abundant nutrients with potent antioxidant properties that protect our cells from damage. It is also a rich source of magnesium, which helps us to relax and generally provides a feel-good factor. Cacao is bitter to taste, which is why sugar is added to commercial chocolate bars and sweets. This is especially a requirement for milk chocolate, to prevent the rancidity of the dairy solids. It is the sugar, not the cacao, that is so addictive, and obviously provides no benefit.

We at Honestly Healthy love cacao – hence the abundance of recipes that include this beneficial ancient ingredient, first discovered in South America thousands of years ago. (See Treats and snacks, page 148 and Desserts, page 168.)

Leave salt to the sea and the Himalayas

Salt was first used to preserve meats and fish in an age when refrigerators hadn't been invented, and when fishermen went to sea for several weeks at a time. This is no longer the case, and we are now fastidious about ensuring that use-by dates are not exceeded and we have the luxury of being able to buy fresh food daily. Most vegetables contain appropriate levels of salt and nutrients (see the tables on pages 16–19), and it should not be necessary to add any or much to your cooking. Use herbs and spices instead to provide additional flavour. Himalayan salt, used in the recipes, is mineral rich and balances sodium with many other vital nutrients, helping to create a better balance in your body, and not posing the threat of dehydration. Most commercially produced salt is processed, stripping out many of the other essential minerals, whereas the salt from the Himalayas is centuries, if not millennia, old.

Cravings for salt usually indicate a deficiency in minerals – especially zinc, which helps to regulate the sensitivity of our taste buds, as well as being vital for strong immunity and to support adrenal function, which regulates our response to stress. This latter point explains why you might opt for salty snacks when you are overtired and stressed – when you would actually be better off having brown rice, quinoa or barley couscous with pumpkin and sunflower seeds to boost zinc stores.

Good fizz, bad fizz

Real champagne from Champagne in France has had nothing added to it to make it fizzy – the fermentation method and the way the bottles are turned create the bubbles. The bubbles you find in cans of cola are purely synthetic, created by a cocktail of chemicals and aeration. How this behaves in the body is to affect the nervous system, pepping you up artificially, with the inevitable subsequent drop in energy as your blood-sugar levels are again disrupted. *The only natural ingredient in a can of cola is water!* Why not have naturally carbonated water with a few slices of ginger, a stick of lemongrass or a sprig of fresh mint leaves to pep you up? Adding a pinch of cayenne pepper to water will give you more energy than you need, and supergreen powders including spirulina and chlorella provide the highly bioavailable nutrients your body needs, as well as being very, very alkaline.

Caffeine – good or bad?

While coffee is a natural bean, the caffeine it contains does more harm than good in the long term. *The occasional freshly ground coffee is not disruptive, but daily consumption leaches essential minerals from bones and other tissues in the body to buffer the kidneys in its elimination.* The caffeine added to colas is synthetic and far more damaging, interfering with the nervous system and seratonin/dopamine pathways – it is virtually a depressant when excessively consumed.

Breaking habits

A habit is something you have ground into place simply through repetition, and deciding to break it is nothing more than a choice. The fears of 'how will I feel' or 'how will I manage without' can only be diminished by actually making the decision to stop what is harmful to you by replacing the habit with a better choice. There's no time like the present.

Some foods and drinks are so toxic that ceasing to consume them can cause headaches and some muscle aches and pains, but these last only for a few days and exercising speeds up the process of ridding the body of those damaging chemicals. This is what the Cleanse does – clears your body of toxic residues that end up stored in fat cells and which hinder your performance.

It's All About Upgrading

Upgrading is a term we came up with for motivating our friends and clients to make small but significant changes to their eating habits, one step at a time, rather than thinking of the mountain-like challenge of throwing everything out in one go and having to start sprouting their own seeds on day one.

We like to think of it as the same experience as choosing to upgrade your plane ticket from economy to club – while it might cost you a little more in time and effort, the comfort, health improvements and nourishment you will get from this kind of attention will yield its benefits ten-fold. Good food doesn't necessarily cost more – buying fresh ingredients in local markets ticks several boxes in one go – you are supporting local and specialist farmers rather than endless imports from oversees; you are buying in

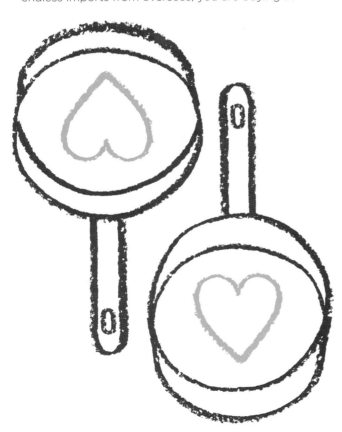

season; you are thinking more carefully about the balance of your foods, and what goes with what – in other words, you are probably buying less and making more out of it.

What to upgrade first?

Upgrading can be done in phases or stages, so that you feel that you are in control of exactly what changes you are making, and being able to perceive the benefits as you go. *Prioritising your specific health complaints, and focusing on those in the first instance will yield huge rewards.* For example, if you frequently suffer from colds and chest infections, chronic rhinitis or other ear, nose and throat problems, it would be best to start with changing your dairy milk intake to nut milks (almond, Brazil nut and macadamia, for example – see pages 53 and 57), soya or feta and halloumi cheeses and soya yogurts, as it is often the whey content of cows' dairy that irritates the mucus lining of the nose, throat and chest endothelial linings. You will observe positive changes literally within days, and your energy levels will build as the stress of the intolerance to the dairy foods dissipates.

On the other hand, if you are suffering from irritable bowel syndrome (IBS), bloating and frequent pain or wind in the abdominal cavity, you would be best to cut out all wheat and yeast-based breads, pastas and noodles, as well as biscuits, cakes and such-like. This book is literally full of wheat- and gluten-free recipes in all sections of the recipes, from breakfast pancakes and granola through to chocolate brownies and coconut bread, buckwheat or rice noodles. For most people, even those who don't suffer from IBS or related discomfort, the health benefits of cutting out commercial breads and biscuits, daily sandwiches and pasta will be immeasurable – and worth the effort for all.

Cook yourself healthier

By making some simple swaps (see opposite) you can make super-nutritious food for yourself in minutes. Don't fret about making everything from scratch initially – search out ready-made varieties of the 'improved' option, before going on to making your own.

Simple but Smart Upgrades

From Ready–prepared bottled juices
To Freshly made juices or blended green drinks
Benefits Pulped juices made at home from whole greens, fruits and vegetables contain all the cholesterol-lowering fibre that is stripped away in commercial juicing, as well as retaining the full vitamin content if consumed within one day.

From Ready-prepared smoothies
To Home-made versions with soya or nut milks, fresh fruits and added hemp or flax seed
Benefits The soya or nut milks provide a good level of non-cows' dairy calcium and protein, without the sugars that are often added to the supermarket varieties. Flax and hemp seeds provide extra essential fatty acids that benefit the nervous system, memory and skin and regulate hormones.

From Ready-prepared muesli, yogurt and granola
To Nutty granola and berries (see page 56)
Benefits Soaking the oats for the muesli activates the enzyme content of the grain, raising the protein content and making it more easily digested and absorbed, plus it has a lower glycaemic index.

From Ready-prepared soups
To Home-made soups with added pulses
Benefits Countless! Far higher mineral and vitamin content, variety and alkalinity – home-made soups allow for using up the stray vegetables from other recipes, as well as the increased protein content from beans and pulses, usually only found in very low content in supermarket-bought versions.

From Ready-prepared lasagne or moussaka
To Home-made vegetable bake
Benefits Fresher vegetables and no salt or other additives required to 'hold' a commercial version together for appearance. Home-made allows you to create your own topping – crushed nuts, oats and seeds make delicious and nutritious toppings.

From Ready-prepared pasta-based salads
To Home-made quinoa, brown rice or buckwheat-noodle-based salad or mixed grain and root vegetable salads with feta or smoked tofu and seeds, nuts and other toppings
Benefits The minerals in the home-cooked wholegrain quinoa and buckwheat are far higher than commercially produced pasta, and these grains do not cause bloating.

From Ready-made salad dressings
To Selection of fresh, home-made dressings to store in the fridge
Benefits Nothing beats a fresh dressing for flavour and variety. Commercial versions contain additives, sugar and salt to give them a long shelf life.

From Tea and coffee
To Fresh root ginger, lemongrass, fennel and peppermint teas; dandelion root or chicory coffee granules (available in all good wholefood stores)
Benefits Stimulating fresh ingredients that naturally give you a lift, without the subsequent come-down that caffeine provides. No anxiety and no cellulite (caffeine is stored in fatty tissues and is a known cause of orange-peel thighs and bottoms).

From Sliced white bread or croissants
To Commercial rye bread or pumpernickel, sunflower or pumpkin-seed flatbreads; home-made rye soda bread or coconut bread (see page 60), buckwheat wraps and pancakes
Benefits Omitting commerically produced yeast breads lowers your intake of sugars and salt. Wholegrain breads have a far higher vitamin and mineral content. Tastier, and far more satisfying.

From Ready-prepared puddings
To Home-made ice creams or cakes
Benefits No sugars or addictive additives. Packed with fresh fruits and nut milks for protein. Unbeatable versus unbearable – no contest!

The Honestly Healthy Cleanse

Many consider cleansing to be something the body does naturally, by itself – which indeed it does. However, with the total toxic load of the commercially produced foods we consume, drinks we imbibe and airborne chemicals we are exposed to on a daily basis, it is little wonder that we need to address this toxicity in a more strenuous way several times a year.

When to embark on a Cleanse

At Honestly Healthy, we recommend carrying out a Cleanse with the change of the seasons – when the temperature changes and your body is adapting to this. The body is designed to adapt to seasonal changes.

To be clear, the Cleanse is *not* what others call a detox. Our bodies are eliminating through urine, faeces and sweat on a moment-to-moment basis, and the liver has its own complex detoxification system. However, the Cleanse *is* a way of supporting your body's natural systems in these processes, by providing nutrient-dense drinks and foods that are all known to have elimination-enhancing properties.

How long should you Cleanse for?

You can choose to run your Cleanse for as long as you want between five days and three weeks, depending on how much you want to change your eating habits. For your first Cleanse, aim for seven to ten days and see how you feel. If you are bounding with energy (which we are pretty sure you will be), then continue for a further week, before moving on to the Lifestyle phase of the programme (see page 38).

The first stage of the Cleanse is to remove all those foods and drinks you have been consuming in a regular or addictive pattern (see What's your fix?, page 27), to lighten the load on your digestive system. If coffee is your drug of choice, you will be going without; if a pain au chocolat is your morning fix, you will quickly notice how different you feel without it.

Cooking methods for the Cleanse

Steaming, stir-steaming ('frying' food at a lower temperature with water to create steam), gently simmering and, best of all, raw and/or marinated in lemon juice and olive oil are the preferred cooking methods for all vegetables, as these are most nutritious. During the Cleanse, avoid stir-frying, baking or roasting vegetables as higher temperatures can lower the overall nutrition of a dish.

Preparing to embark on your Cleanse

Plan your Cleanse by ensuring that you will have plenty of time to relax and will not have to attend business functions and parties, where you are unlikely to be able to find the correct foods and may be tempted into eating the foods you know are not recommended. Ideally, you want to have time for light daily exercise – yoga and pilates, swimming and dance are all perfect as they involve using all the body muscle groups, and in particular stimulate the digestion to help eliminate toxins more efficiently.

Allocating time to ensure you have sufficient foods in your fridge on a daily basis is the key to the success of the Cleanse. Follow the menu planner (see page 36) to start with, so you know what you are having each day. You will not go hungry if you aim to eat every two to three hours – a juice, smoothie, soup or salad – for the first two days. Thereafter, you can space out your consumption to every three to four hours, as your body is absorbing highly bioavailable nutrients from your meals. Keep your fluid intake high to minimise cravings for the first few days.

The benefits of being more alkaline will start to appear within a matter or days. *You will be able to think more clearly, sleep more soundly, have greater levels of energy and concentration than you have had for some time. Your skin will brighten, your eyes will sparkle and there will be a new spring in your step.* Internally, your immune system will respond by clearing out old ills – viruses may reappear, but not for long, as the immune army will start to strengthen, and you will feel fitter than you have for a long time.

Repeating the Cleanse up to four times in the first year, as the seasons change, is ideal. After the Cleanse, you can move on to the Lifestyle phase, expanding the variety of foods you can eat and choosing from a vast array of recipes in the second part of this book. Enjoy!

Foods to avoid during the Cleanse

We recommend cutting out the following altogether during your Cleanse:

Red meat, chicken, turkey, duck, all eggs, fish and shellfish
Reason These foods are predominantly acid-forming and can take 2–4 days to go through your digestive tract – we are aiming for fast-moving foods to cleanse your system.

Most dairy produce (goat's milk and cheese, ewe's halloumi and feta are included in the Lifestyle, but NOT on the Cleanse)
Reason Acid-forming, and most animal-based dairy produce is mucus-forming in the respiratory and digestive tracts, which interferes with nutrient absorption.

Coffee, tea, cola drinks, fizzy water
Reason All acid-forming and a stress to the adrenal glands; also inhibit nutrient absorption. Contain tannins and artificial colourings, which often contribute to headaches and migraines. Carbonated waters are often high in sodium.

Sugar in any form
Reason Acid-forming and produces blood-sugar highs and lows, creating artificial bursts of energy followed by fatigue. Also feeds pathogenic bacteria in the gut, which cause wind, bloating, fatigue, headaches, muscle aches and pains.

All breads, cakes and biscuits containing gluten-flour (wheat, oats, rye and barley)
Reason While oats, rye and barley are all highly nutritious grains in their own right, they do contain gluten – the protein portion of the grain – which tends to create a 'sticky' mass in an already bunged-up digestive tract. Beneficial grains are important during the Lifestyle, but not during the Cleanse.

Couscous, semolina, spelt (all wheat-based grains)
Reason Highest gluten-containing grain, prevents cleansing through the digestive system.

Lentils, oats, peanut butter, kidney beans, chickpeas
Reason Low-alkaline and slow to digest. These are all beneficial during the Lifestyle but NOT on the Cleanse.

All commercial breakfast cereals
Reason Over-processed, high in sugars, salt and other additives. Burden on kidneys to break down chemicals.

All rice (brown, red and basmati)
Reason Slow to move through the digestive tract.

All take-away and convenience foods
Reason Excessive additives and over-processing place additional burden on the digestive tract to 'break down' the foreign items contained in such foods.

All packet snacks
Reason Deep-fried and salted, they stimulate the kidneys to work overtime, dehydrating the body and unbalancing the minerals sodium and potassium.

All condiments – for example, tomato ketchup, sauces, vinegars, mustard and pickles
Reason Acid-forming and unbalancing the minerals sodium and potassium.

Alcohol – including all wines, spirits and fermented after-dinner drinks and digestifs
Reason All alcohol is sugar-forming in the gut and disruptive to the body's natural blood-sugar regulation. Alcohol stimulates sugar and carbohydrate cravings, as well as interfering with nutrient absorption.

Foods to enjoy during the Cleanse

The majority of foods that you will be consuming are vegetable-based, as these are rich in nutrients that support cleansing at a cellular level, as well as providing the fibre required to clean the digestive tract thoroughly. *These may all be eaten raw or cooked, but the closer to their natural state they are, the more intact and undisturbed the nutrients will be.*

Dark green leafy vegetables

Curly kale, Savoy cabbage, spinach, rocket, watercress, parsley, coriander leaf, summer and winter greens and broccoli are excellent in juices (see Cleansing juices, page 37, and Green smoothies, page 46), with salads and simply steamed vegetables as part of a meal.

The allium family of vegetables

Known for their cleansing and liver-supporting properties, onions, leeks, garlic and spring onions all contain the amino acid L-cysteine, upon which the liver is dependent for safely clearing certain foods and toxic substances. Steaming onions, leeks and garlic sweetens them, and adding them raw to juices and smoothies packs a huge immune-supporting punch.

Supergreens

Much is written about the power of the microscopic blue-green algae found in the untainted Klamath Lakes in Oregon, USA, which some believe hold the only toxin-free waters left on the planet. This algae is possibly the richest source of vegetarian nutrients to be found, and many have fasted for several days drinking these living algae and water alone.

At Honestly Healthy we don't advise that you go to such drastic measures, but we do encourage you to have ½ teaspoon of powdered algae dissolved in 0.5–1 litre (17–35fl oz/2–4 cups) water per day, either combined with other juices or as a stand-alone drink. The higher the concentration of algae to water, the richer the nutrient shot – try it and see for yourself.

Sprouted beans and seeds

By far the most nutrient-dense options during the Cleanse, adding sprouts to your daily regime will provide you with the best protein/vitamin/mineral combinations, and these 'living foods' will have you bursting with energy. Remember to dress them only with olive oil or nut/seed oils, such as walnut, hazelnut or pumpkin seed, together with lemon or lime juice, but no vinegars. Choose organic varieties that are fresh and green (avoid any that have gone brown at the tips). Best of all, buy a stack of sprouting trays and sprout your own – always so satisfying. The best beans to sprout are mung, soya, alfalfa, lentils and split peas.

Fruits

The only fruits recommended during the Cleanse are apples, lemons, grapefruits and limes as these are the most alkalising. Some avocados can be included, as these provide excellent protein, vitamin E and essential fats, but should not be eaten every day as they are rich.

Apples support the liver and gall bladder in their inherent cleansing roles. Add whole apples to juices to provide a little sweetness, if you like, and also for their pectin, contained just under their skin, which helps to latch onto toxins in the gut and remove them with the additional fibre. All other fruits, including berries, should be reserved for the Lifestyle phase.

Spirulina

Considered to be as potent as blue-green algae (see Supergreens, opposite), spirulina is one of the smallest single-cell plants, packed with iron and B vitamins, including B12 (very important for vegetarians, as this essential B vitamin is often lacking in their diet). Research has found that the immune-boosting and liver-cleansing properties of spirulina are superb and multi-faceted, so adding a teaspoon of the dried powdered variety to your juices and cold soups is well worth it! Do not heat spirulina, as the nutrients are easily damaged in such a microscopic entity.

Sea vegetables

Seaweeds, such as wakame, kelp, nori and kombu, are all alkalising, and contain calcium, potassium and iron. They are considered essential in the macrobiotic approach to eating – introduced to the West some 50 years ago by Japanese Michio Kushi. The macrobiotic approach takes vegetarianism to an extreme and can be difficult to adhere to in everyday life, as it is hugely time-consuming to prepare. For the Honestly Healthy Cleanse, you can buy some of these seaweeds fresh, but soaking dried varieties and adding them to juices, smoothies and soups is beneficial, as they are known to remove toxins rapidly and settle the digestion.

Dairy alternatives

While several nut milks (see pages 53 and 57) are favoured in the Lifestyle part of the Honestly Healthy programme, only almond milk is recommended during the Cleanse, as it is really alkaline and contains an abundance of magnesium, which is relaxing to body and mind and encourages more rapid movement of foods through the digestive tract. Making your own almond milk takes only a little time and is preferable to commercial varieties, which are often sweetened. When choosing soya milk look for organic varieties. Rice milk is *not* suitable for the Cleanse, although you can use it occasionally in the Lifestyle phase, providing the milk is derived from brown rather than white rice.

Hemp seed, flax seed and pea protein powders

Nowadays these protein-rich ground seeds and peas are all readily available in most supermarkets. The essential fatty acids found in hemp seed and flax seed (linseed) are potently anti-inflammatory and add considerable mineral value to juices and soups. They can also be added to soya-based smoothies for rebuilding and repair, as their zinc, calcium and magnesium content are excellent.

Herbal teas

As most of the Cleanse period involves drinking juices and soups and eating predominantly raw food salads, it is vital to ensure you drink plenty of fluids to help you stay hydrated. Stimulating teas such as ginger and fennel are excellent for supporting the liver's natural cleansing. We recommend that you have a rotation of about four or five teas daily, so you do not over-stimulate any of the cleansing organs unnecessarily. Remember that hot water with lemon or lime is by far the most alkalising of all hot drinks, and making a pot to provide three or four cups first thing in the morning is ideal to get your digestive system moving beautifully. Do not drink either green or white teas on the Cleanse, but save these slightly caffeinated, yet highly antioxidant varieties for the Lifestyle phase instead.

Menu Planner for the Cleanse Phase

DAY 1
Morning
Lemon and hot water on rising
The Ultimate Morning Wake-up smoothie (page 47)
Quinoa Porridge with Macadamia Nut Milk (page 53)

Lunch
Falafel Wraps with salsa and yogurt (page 70)

Snack
Spinach and Chickpea Hummus with Raw Flax Seed Crackers (page 167)

Dinner
Mixed Vegetable and Soya Bean Hotpot (page 82)

DAY 2
Morning
Lemon and hot water on rising
Toxin Reducer juice (page 37)
American-style Buckwheat Pancakes (page 52) (without the blackberry compote) but with soya yogurt

Lunch
Dill Steamed Artichokes (page 75) with a fresh green salad

Snack
Beetroot and Walnut Dip (page 166) with gluten-free crackers

Dinner
Fennel and Pear Soup (page 80)

DAY 3
Morning
Lemon and hot water on rising
Liver Love juice (page 37)
Raw Buckwheat and Cinnamon Granola (page 54) with Almond Milk (page 57)

Lunch
Watercress, Roasted Onion and Pistachio Salad (page 88)

Snack
Smoky Aubergine Dip (page 166) with fresh vegetable crudités

Dinner
Layered Vegetable Bake (page 112)

DAY 4
Morning
Lemon and hot water on rising
Fresh smoothie (page 46)
Nutty Granola (page 56) with Almond Milk (page 57)

Lunch
Spicy Tofu Skewers (page 124) and Mint-and-Mango Marinated Courgette Spaghetti (page 126)

Snack
'Cheesy' Kale Chips (page 159)

Dinner
Portobello Mushroom and Fennel Salad (page 100)

DAY 5
Morning
Lemon and hot water on rising
Hydrator juice (page 37)
Avocado on Toast (page 49) with a poached egg

Lunch
Butternut Squash Soup (page 79)

Snack
Nut butter (page 160) with raw crudités

Dinner
Tomato and Mushroom Dhal (page 127) with Sweet Tomato Tabbouleh (page 146)

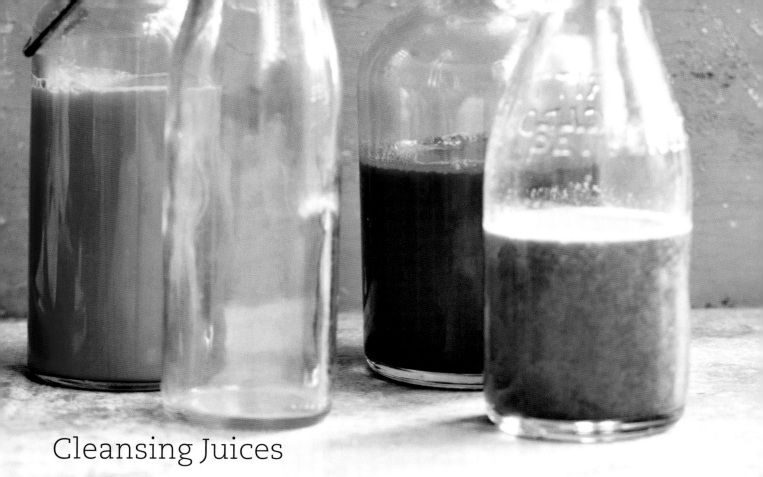

Cleansing Juices

The importance of hydration cannot be overestimated during the Cleanse phase. The recipes below contain a wide variety of nutrients that support liver, kidneys and bowel to clear the backlog of toxins you have accumulated. They help to keep energy up and sugar cravings down.

Toxin Reducer
♥♥♥

1 fennel
½ cucumber (or 1 small)
2.5cm/1in piece of fresh root ginger
juice of ½ lemon squeezed in
1 green apple

Liver Love
♥♥♥

1 large beetroot (beet)
2 handfuls of spinach
3 carrots
½ handful of flat-leaf parsley

Hydrator
♥♥♥

1 handful of broccoli
1 pear
2 celery sticks
1 sprig of mint

Immune Booster
♥♥♥

3 beetroot (beet)
2 red apples
2.5cm/1in piece of fresh root ginger
juice of ½ lemon squeezed in

Green Goddess
♥♥♥

2 apples
1 handful of kale
½ cucumber
1 handful of watercress

To make any of these juices, simply put through a juicer.

The Honestly Healthy Lifestyle

Having completed the Cleanse phase, you will now understand what it's like to think more clearly, have more energy, wake up feeling refreshed and have the motivation to take on board the principles described earlier (see Know your good groups, page 12, and Learn new eating habits, page 20).

At Honestly Healthy, we don't say you have to aspire to eating in perfect balance 100% of the time – instead, we encourage you to look to nourishing yourself most of the time, as you already know how much better you feel for taking out so much of the rubbish that has made up the majority of your food and drink consumption over the last few years. Whether you are restricted for time, money or locally sourced fresh ingredients, you need to make a commitment to your own health and take responsibility for helping to make the improvements happen.

Kitchen equipment

We recommend that you equip your kitchen with all the right tools to make your life easier. You don't have to buy all this equipment in one go, but you do need to collect the essentials over time. Wait for sales to come up for the more expensive pieces (food processor, Vitamix blender, juicer) or check out eBay for those items that others have been given and simply never used. All this equipment is for your ease of preparation and can be hugely time-saving. A visit to a good kitchen shop or catering outlet will inspire you to become your own chef-at-home!

- Food processor
- Vitamix blender (the best) or other good-quality, strong-blade blender
- Juicer (Braun, Waring, Phillips)
- Hand-held blender (great for soups and dips before you make a bigger investment)
- Mandolin
- Good set of knives
- Chopping boards
- Slow-cooker
- Dehydrator
- Spiraliser

STOCKING UP

The first important move is to make sure that you have all you need in your kitchen. Being prepared is the key!

Your stock of dry goods and herbs and spices is the foundation of a well-prepared healthy kitchen, allowing you to create a meal at the drop of a hat, with simply the addition of some fresh ingredients.

Include the following in your store cupboard and you will be able to create most of the recipes found in this book:

- Chickpeas, butter beans, black-eyed beans, pinto beans, red kidney beans
- Red and brown lentils, puy lentils, black beluga lentils, dhal red lentils, yellow split peas
- Pearl barley, brown rice, red Camargue rice, black rice noodles, buckwheat noodles
- Dried wakame, nori and dulse seaweeds and bonito flakes
- Dried fruits for soaking in Bircher muesli – apricots, cranberries, goji berries, sultanas and raisins
- Cumin, turmeric, mustard seed, cinnamon, nutmeg, allspice, bay leaves, coriander seed, fenugreek seed, cumin seed, black and red peppercorns, paprika, cayenne pepper, sumac
- Agave syrup, Sweet Freedom syrup, manuka honey, xylitol, yacon syrup
- Cashews, almonds, hazelnuts, pecans, walnuts (store in fridge for freshness)
- Almond nut, hazelnut and cashew nut butters and tahini (should also be kept in fridge once opened or made)
- Coconut butter and coconut milk
- Cacao powder and cacao butter
- Apple cider vinegar, balsamic vinegar, Braggs Aminos, tamari (wheat-free soy sauce), mirin (rice wine)

Cooking methods for the Lifestyle

All the methods used in the Cleanse (see page 33) also apply to the Lifestyle phase of the programme, with the inclusion of sautéing vegetables, tofu and grains in the early part of their cooking. Sautéing allows oils to be used to cook the food at a lower temperature than frying, to soften the food, without overcooking or damaging the nutrients contained therein.

Healing herbs and spices

It's a good idea to choose recipes that use one, two or more of these fantastic healing herbs and spices. You'll enjoy their benefits in no time.

Turmeric

Our number one favourite ingredient – *this ancient spice has been used in Ayurvedic medicine in India for over 3,000 years to boost the natural killer cells of the immune system, warding off infections, protecting against viruses and may prevent the development of cancers.* Its yellow colouring is effected by the curcuminoids, an inherent healing compound in both turmeric and cumin, which are anti-inflammatory and stimulating to the liver and gall bladder in their natural detoxification processes.

Ginger

Also a favourite for us, we prefer to use fresh root ginger, but dried ginger powder is also beneficial. This root vegetable also stimulates the liver to flush out toxins, helps with both morning and motion sickness, has been found to help lower cholesterol and high blood pressure, and is a marvellous tonic for the skin. *We love adding ginger to green smoothies, breads, salads and main dishes to pep up the flavour and add a spring to your step*.

Chilli peppers

Again, we encourage using fresh when you can, but wouldn't discourage dried chillies either. The heat of the chilli comes from a compound called capsaicin, which is found in a lesser amount in bell peppers. *Capsaicin stimulates metabolism, supports thyroid function, helps curb carb cravings and encourages good digestion and elimination.* Use carefully, and avoid at night if you are a light sleeper, as chillies will make you dream more vividly!

Garlic

Many of our dishes include garlic (both fresh and dried powdered), *as its healing properties are boundless – antibacterial, antiviral, anti-parasitic and liver-supporting*, no healthy kitchen should be without garlic. The amino acid cysteine, which helps the liver in its detox processes, is the main healing component.

Sumac

Few people had heard of sumac until a few years ago, and yet it has been used for millennia to add spice and tartness to raw and cooked dishes, and is slightly sour to taste on its own. It is derived from a berry (*Rhus coriaria*), and grown in the Middle East and Italy. *Sumac stimulates the digestive enzymes in the mouth* (ptyalin) that help to break down dense proteins such as nuts, soy produce and beans, and pulses.

Mustard seeds

Rather than using mustard from a jar, which has vinegar, sugar and sometimes additives, *the humble mustard seed has a lot to offer.* It adds fabulous flavour to salads and soups, while stimulating stomach acid production to ensure you digest your food more efficiently. It is also a rich source of selenium to boost metabolism and immunity.

Meal planning

We have provided you with over 100 recipes in this book to stimulate your palate and cooking skills. None of them are difficult to prepare and, in fact, you will be surprised by how quick and easy most of them are. However, we suggest you start with just two or three days' worth of recipes for breakfast, lunch and dinner, with a couple of snacks, so as not to feel overwhelmed. On the contrary, once you have shopped for the ingredients for those days, you will have more confidence to incorporate this into your Lifestyle.

This is exactly how Natasha started, with her Fridge Fill service to her clients – supplying menus on a Sunday evening and cooking all the dishes on Monday to deliver for the next three days' worth of meals.

Start on a Sunday

If you are working full-time, we suggest you do all your shopping and cooking for the first three days on a Sunday, so that you don't have to think about what to cook for the first half of the week.

Remember that fresh food should be exactly that – *fresh*. Don't be tempted to bulk-buy fruit and vegetables unless you plan to bulk-cook and freeze portions of soups and casseroles! This is not a bad idea when you embark on the Lifestyle, so that you can stay 'on programme'. However, you will soon see how satisfying, quick and easy it is to prepare certain things daily, and we really encourage that all the fresh juices, smoothies and salads are prepared at the time of consuming, for maximum benefit.

Snacking is positively encouraged

We have devoted a proportionately high amount of the recipes – both sweet and savoury – to mini-meals and snacks, as this is an area where so many who are aiming to eat healthily fall down. Know that most commercially produced nut-and-seed bars are often

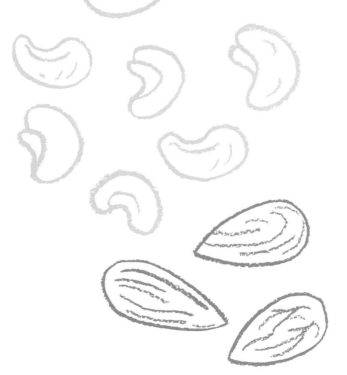

laden with sugar to prevent the bars from going rancid, and you will be far better off making your own (see Granola Bars, page 150, or Sticky Seed Flapjacks, page 152). Similarly, many commercial dips and spreads have high levels of salt and additives to prevent browning or rancidity. *When you see that it literally takes five minutes to prepare your own hummus (see Spinach and chickpea hummus, page 167) and you have plenty of celery, carrots, mangetout (snow peas) and cucumbers in the fridge, you have ready-made alkaline snacks at your fingertips.* Even Avocado on Toast (see page 49) takes mere moments and is so satisfying, as the balance of protein to carbohydrates provides you with a perfect balance of slow-release energy.

Taking food when you travel

Whether you're travelling by road, rail, boat or plane, the foods on offer at available cafés, bakeries and delis are usually high-fat, high-sugar, high-salt and therefore high-acid. This will simply leave you dehydrated, and yearning for more of the same.

Avoid these eventualities by being prepared – you can't take your own green juice on a plane, but you can take a bag of sprouted beans and seeds and those little pearls of protein will stave off hunger for hours! Similarly, if you know you have a car journey of several hours, bake some Coconut Bread (see page 160) or Chocolate Coconut Balls (see page 156), some Granola Bars (see page 150) or some dips and crudités (see pages 166–67), and make a batch of fresh vegetable juice to take in a thermos to preserve its freshness. *You will arrive at your destination perky and bright-eyed* as opposed to tired, irritable and bloated!

Energy through the day

In a world where we are becoming increasingly overwhelmed and overburdened with our responsibilities, multi-tasking and frequent travel, prioritising *when* to eat is key. Too often, meals and snacks are 'put off' in favour of 'just finishing this before I eat'. *In the Lifestyle, we encourage you to plan your day around when you eat, rather than the other way round.* In France and some other European countries, as well as China and Japan, large corporations have prioritised feeding their employees regularly

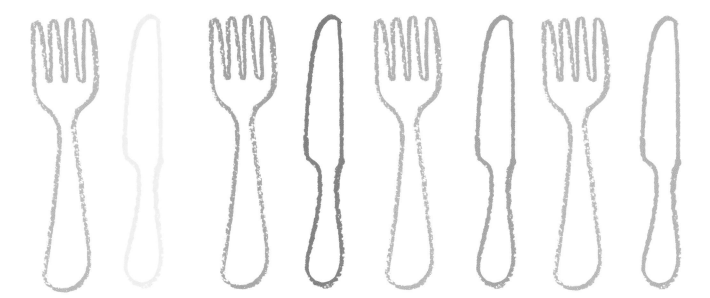

throughout the day as they know how this will affect productivity within the business. For many, especially those who work for themselves, this discipline simply isn't implemented. So, we recommend allocating a midday lunchtime, and start by setting an alarm on your watch or phone. *Moving away from your desk or other work station for half an hour at least to have a midday meal will more than double your productivity in the ensuing three hours.* Those who 'skip' meals simply lower their productivity measurably. Additionally, if you are someone who works late into the evening, taking time for a late-afternoon high-protein snack (Beetroot and Walnut Dip, see page 166) or mini-meal (Falafel Wraps with salsa and yogurt, see page 70) ensures that your blood-sugar levels remain balanced, your concentration and focus sharp and that the extra hours you put in are worth every minute.

Eating for exercise

Some like to exercise first thing in the morning, others at lunchtime and the rest after work (or not at all!). As well as toning the body, exercise raises endorphins, which stimulate serotonin production – the 'happy and contented' neurotransmitter that is received in both the brain, where it increases motivation, and the digestive system (sometimes known as the 'second

brain'), where it produces feelings of calm and satisfaction. *It is no coincidence that the CEOs of both small and large businesses are the primary high-level exercisers.* They know the value of endorphins and serotonin production and of the feel-good factor and sense of being in control that goes with that.

Morning exercisers

If you are a runner and you choose to run in the morning, do not eat anything solid before you run – a good high-protein shake is what you need (see Smoothies, pages 46–48). Including soya or almond milk (see Milks, page 57), hemp or flax seed, almonds, cashews and walnuts all add both protein and essential fats to your pre-workout drink. Anything more solid is likely to repeat on you when running. Post-run food should be eaten within half an hour and should be a good balance of protein, essential fats and carbohydrate, for example Raw Buckwheat and Cinnamon Granola with fresh berries (see page 54).

Working out at lunchtime

If you exercise in your lunch hour, make sure to have a complex carbohydrate snack mid-morning, such as spelt or rye bread with a dip of your choice. This will ensure you have adequate glucose stores in the muscles to take you through your workout without leaving you feeling totally exhausted. Eating a well-balanced lunch mid-afternoon will balance your blood-sugar levels and ensure that you maintain focus and energy through the afternoon's work.

Exercising at the end of the day

For evening exercisers, you need a second mini-lunch (or more of the same from your first meal), to provide you with sufficient energy for your workout, and to prepare something satisfying for when you get home in the evening. *Soups provide a great balance of energy-fuelling complex carbohydrates and proteins; include pearl barley, quinoa and buckwheat, with a vast array of seasonal vegetables to ensure ample antioxidants to mop up the free radicals produced in your workout.* You may either take a thermos flask with you to work, or know that you have a slow-cooked meal waiting for you when you get home.

For those who choose yoga as their primary form of exercise, remember that it is important not to eat for a couple of hours prior to your practice, as many of the asanas work directly on the digestive tract as a whole, and eating solid foods will cause discomfort. Drinking vegetable juices up to half an hour prior to your practice is preferable.

And for those who are not exercising at all – *get moving*! Lack of exercise is acid-forming in the body, promoting lack of energy and depression. Research has confirmed this fact time and again – hence the saying 'eat with your body in mind', to which we always advocate moving your body. Lack of exercise leads to shallow breathing, which is also acid-forming, preventing the removal of natural toxins from the body. Whatever you choose to do, from dance to kick-boxing, running, riding or swimming – just do it! Exercise is the number one stress-buster, and stress is the number one cause of disease.

Managing stress through food

It has been shown through much research that stress leads to increased production of cortisol, a hormone released from the adrenal glands in response to our 'fight or flight' response mechanism in the body. Acute stress is manageable, and the adrenal glands have been designed to help rebalance our reaction to fright, surprise, shock and immediate reactions for our survival. *However, chronic stress is depleting to the adrenals, and subsequently the thyroid gland (found at the base of the neck, just below your Adam's apple), as well as being highly acid-forming to the body.* This is why those who are under constant pressure at work, or caring for another family member constantly, or experiencing financial difficulties, regularly get sick. This is your body's way of telling you to take more care of yourself and prioritise your own health. This is a time when the alkaline approach is paramount, as your body is producing much acid, inflammation and the precursors for serious disease. Think how often you have heard a friend saying, 'I think I need to change my lifestyle – I can feel that there is something seriously wrong with me.'

Don't wait for the seriously wrong to happen – take charge of your own health *now*, and embark on the Honestly Healthy Alkaline Programme. You won't regret it, and you'll enjoy the benefits of feeling really well for the first time in years. Your energy will soar, your weight will balance itself to the weight you are supposed to be and you will feel years younger within a matter of months.

We want you to have the benefits we have both found through living our lives this way – we know how easy it is to eat Honestly Healthily, because we do it ourselves. As they say, the proof of the pudding is in the eating, so get cooking in your kitchen and see for yourself. You can have the treats as well as all the greens, because we've made sure that they nourish you in the best way. *Eat with your body in mind.*

Menu Planner for the Lifestyle Phase

DAY 1
Morning
Nutty Granola with a nut milk (pages 56–57)
A Green Smoothie (pages 46–47)

Lunch
Spanish Omelette with Dill and Sweet Potato (page 110) with a simple green leaf salad or Pulsed Broad Bean and Pearl Barley Salad (page 99)

Snack
Beetroot and Walnut Dip (page 166) with Raw Flax Seed Crackers (page 167)

Evening
Thai Yellow Curry with Brown Rice (page 142)

DAY 2
Morning
Scrambled Eggs and Portobello Mushroom with Melted Goat's Cheese (page 60)
Toxin Reducer juice (page 37)

Lunch
Sweetcorn and Broad Bean Fritters with a Feta, Cucumber and Spinach Salad (pages 122–123)

Snack
Handful of almonds, soaked

Evening
Mixed Vegetable and Soya Bean Hotpot (page 82) with Sweet Potato Bread toast (page 162)

Dessert
Raw Chocolate Mousse (page 170)

DAY 3
Morning
Avocado on Toast (page 49)
Mango Coconut smoothie (page 48)

Lunch
Butternut Squash Soup (page 79)

Snack
Smoky Aubergine Dip (page 166) with crudités

Evening
Caramelised Pear and Lentil Salad (page 94)

DAY 4
Morning
Nut and Berry Layered Breakfast (page 55)
Green Goddess juice (page 37)

Lunch
Quinoa and Cranberry Burgers (page 116) with Pomegranate and Mozzarella Salad (page 98)

Snack
'Cheesy' Kale Chips (page 159)

Evening
Red Rice and Beetroot Risotto (page 130)
Sweet-potato Chocolate Brownie (page 174)

DAY 5
Morning
American-style Buckwheat Pancakes with Blackberry Compote (page 52)

Lunch
Dill Steamed Artichoke (page 75) with a serving of Roots and Walnut Salad (page 98)

Snack
Spinach and Chickpea Hummus (page 167) with raw crudités

Evening
Noodle and Smoked Tofu Salad with Mirin Dressing (page 121)
Raw Mango Coconut Balls (page 156)

breakfasts

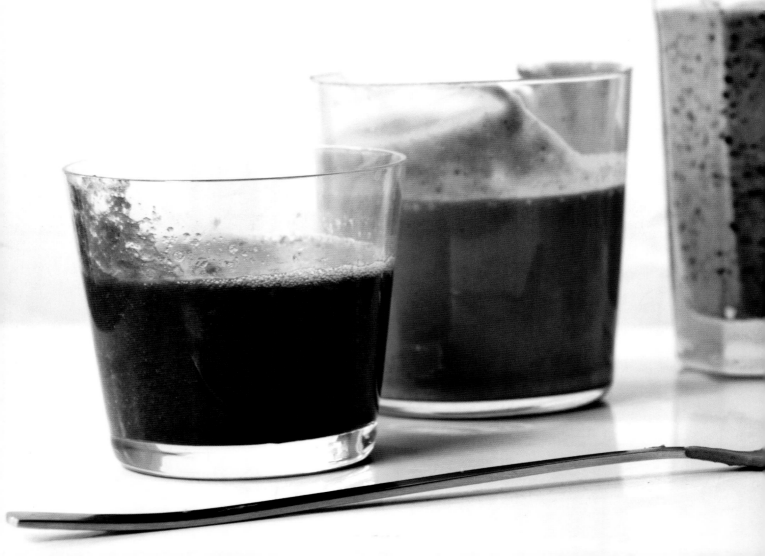

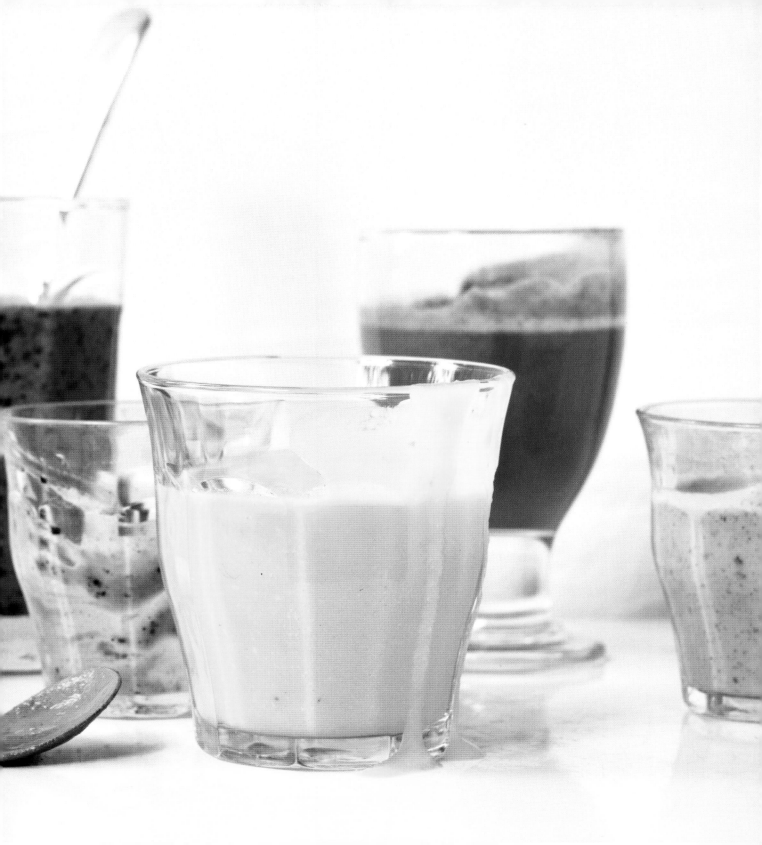

Green Smoothies

A green smoothie isn't a juice, but a mixture of water, leafy greens and fruits, thoroughly blended together. The blender breaks down the cellulose structure in the greens, thereby unlocking their valuable nutrients. You can change the fruit to whatever you like and add extra ingredients as you wish, so play around with flavours. Use about 40% greens to 60% fruit to start, plus just enough water to run the blender and create the thickness you like best. Smoothies are fast and easy to make and will complement any diet or lifestyle.

To make any of these smoothies, simply blend the ingredients in a Vitamix or high-speed blender until smooth. **All smoothies serve 2**

Fresh

1 ripe pear, cored and chopped
1 bunch of kale
sprig of mint
250ml (8fl oz/1 cup) purified or filtered
    water
250ml (8fl oz/1 cup) apple juice

Hydrating Sweet Fix

1 soft ripe peach
1 banana
30g (1¼oz) baby spinach leaves
1 tsp agave syrup
250ml (8fl oz/1 cup) coconut water

Cold Buster

1 bunch of pak choi, roughly chopped
1 banana
125g (4oz/scant 1 cup) frozen raspberries
125g (4oz/generous ¾ cup) frozen
   blueberries
350ml (12fl oz/1⅓ cups) purified or
   filtered water

Spicy

1 handful of spinach
125g (4oz/generous ¾ cup) frozen
   blueberries
1 ripe pear, cored and chopped
½ ripe banana
1 tsp grated fresh root ginger
250ml (8fl oz/1 cup) purified or filtered
   water

THINGS TO ADD...
Probiotic powder
Omega oils (we love Udo's)
Raw flax seeds
Spirulina
Wheatgrass
Maca
Lúcuma (sweet-tasting)
Hemp protein powder
   (quite earthy-tasting, be warned)
Or add your 'supergreens' powder
   instead of individually adding
   all the supergreens.

The Ultimate Morning Wake-up

1 head of pak choi, roughly chopped
½ papaya
½ mango
125ml (4fl oz/½ cup) purified or filtered
   water
250ml (8fl oz/1 cup) coconut water
1 tbsp ground raw flax seeds
1 tsp spirulina powder or any
   'supergreens' powder
2 probiotic capsules (pull the capsule
   apart and tip out the contents)
1 tbsp Udo's oil

Skin Booster

10cm (4in) piece of cucumber,
   roughly chopped
1 handful of spinach
Juice of 1 lemon
2 celery sticks, roughly chopped
1 kiwi
¼ avocado
475ml (16fl oz/scant 2 cups) purified or
   filtered water

TIPS
- Coconut water can be added instead of water.
- Add agave syrup to sweeten if not quite sweet enough.

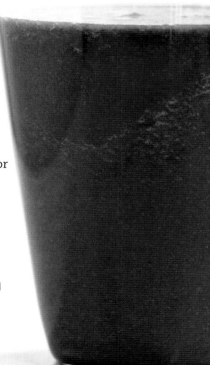

Fruit Smoothies

Nothing can beat these smoothies, complete with cholesterol-lowering fibre, energy-giving complex carbohydrates and protein for building and repair.

Mango Coconut

⅓ mango, sliced

1 banana

475ml (16fl oz/scant 2 cups) coconut water

40g (1½oz/½ cup) dessicated coconut (dry unsweetened shredded coconut)

½ tsp vanilla extract

Very Berry

125g (4oz/generous ¾ cup) mixed berries

150g (5oz/scant 1 cup) raw almonds

1 ripe banana

⅛ tsp cinnamon

1–2 tbsp agave syrup (or a few drops of stevia), depending on the ripeness of the berries

Nutty Chocolate

475ml (16fl oz/scant 2 cups) Macadamia Nut Milk (see page 53)

2 very ripe bananas

2 tbsp raw unsweetened cacao powder

1 tsp vanilla extract

2 tbsp agave syrup, or to taste

Blueberry Nut

250ml (8fl oz/1 cup) Hemp Milk (see page 57)

250ml (8fl oz/1 cup) apple juice

2 bananas

250g (8oz/1⅔ cups) blueberries

30g (1¼oz/scant ¼ cup) raw almonds

30g (1¼oz/⅓ cup) raw walnuts

2 tbsp raw flax seeds

Brazilian Berry

125g (4oz/scant 1 cup) strawberries

125g (4oz/scant 1 cup) raspberries

125g (4oz/generous ¾ cup) blueberries

50g (2oz/¼ cup) raw Brazil nuts

750ml (1¼ pints/3 cups) purified or filtered water

2 ice cubes

3 ready-to-eat dried prunes

1 tbsp ground raw flax seeds

¼ tsp cinnamon

Blend the ingredients in a Vitamix or high-speed blender until smooth. **All smoothies serve 2**

Avocado on Toast

serves 1

1 ripe avocado
1 tbsp extra virgin olive oil
Juice of ½ lemon
1 slice of toast (made from any of the bread recipes, see pages 160–163)
Freshly ground black pepper

Super-quick and easy to make, and very nourishing and filling to help you start the day. You can also have this as a mid-afternoon snack to keep you going.

Remove the stone from the avocado and slice lengthways into thin slices. Gently toss the avocado slices in the olive oil and lemon juice. Arrange the avocado slices on the toast. It's as simple as that.

Serve immediately, sprinkled with black pepper.

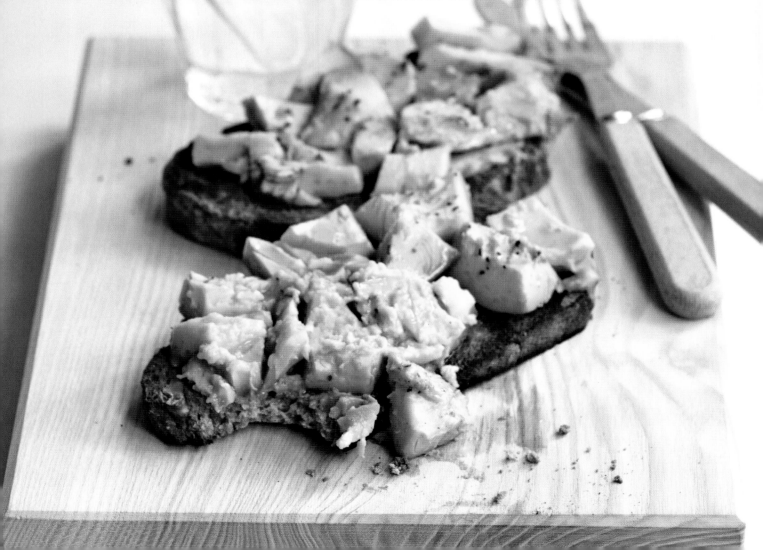

Not all fabulous treats need be bad for you – on the contrary, the macadamia nuts and pomegranate seeds help lower cholesterol, and quinoa is one of the highest protein seeds you can eat.

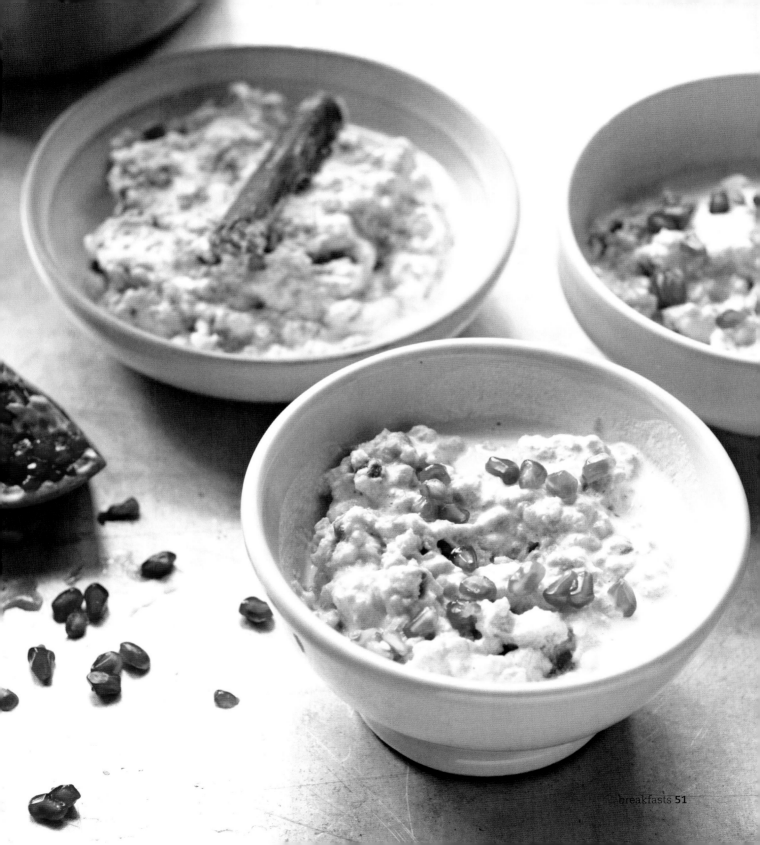

American-style Buckwheat Pancakes

makes 6–8

70g (2¾oz/½ cup) buckwheat
   flour
70g (2¾oz/½ cup) rice flour
1 tsp baking powder
½ tsp Himalayan pink salt
300ml (½ pint/scant 1¼ cups)
   Brown Rice Milk (see page 57)
1 tbsp lemon juice
1 tbsp sunflower oil, plus extra
   for greasing
1 tbsp rice syrup

(Pictured on page 50.) Feeling cosy and indulgent on a weekend? Why not treat yourself to a not-so-naughty breakfast. Feel free to experiment – try adding honey, stewed fruits or even a delicious raw chocolate sauce!

Place the buckwheat flour, rice flour, baking powder and salt in a large bowl and mix well.

Place the milk, lemon juice, sunflower oil and rice syrup in another bowl and mix well, then stir into the dry ingredients and mix gently until just combined, being careful not to overmix.

Wipe a frying pan lightly with oil and heat over a medium heat. Place a poachette ring or pastry ring in the pan and ladle in 1 tablespoon of the pancake mixture. Cook until air bubbles start to appear on the surface of the pancake. Do not turn until this point. Remove the mould, turn the pancake and cook for about 1 minute on the other side, until set. Repeat until all the mixture is used and cooked.

Serve in a stack, layered with Blackberry Compote (see below) and soya yogurt, or with fresh fruit and agave syrup to accompany.

Blackberry Compote

200g (7oz/generous ¾ cup)
   blackberries, rinsed and
   drained
2 tsp water
1 tbsp honey
Pancakes, granola or yogurt, to
   serve

Place the ingredients in a pan over a low heat. Simmer for 10 minutes, stirring occasionally, until the berries are lovely and soft.

Blend the compote until smooth and serve warm or chilled with pancakes, granola or yogurt.

Quinoa Porridge with Macadamia Nut Milk

serves 4

Seeds from 1 pomegranate
200g (7oz/2 cups) quinoa flakes
75g (3oz/scant ⅔ cup) goji berries
1 cinnamon stick
475ml (16fl oz/scant 2 cups) Macadamia Nut Milk (see below)
750ml (1¼ pints/3 cups) water
100g (3½oz/¾ cup) raspberries

(Pictured on page 51.) Macadamia nuts, while more acidic in pH, have abundant essential fats and zinc to boost immunity, while goji berries add the antioxidant beta-carotene. This 'porridge' is higher in protein than the conventional porridge (oatmeal) made with oats.

To remove the seeds from the pomegranate, roll it firmly on a work surface to loosen the seeds, then cut it in half and scoop out the seeds with a teaspoon (or see page 98 for another method). Set aside while you make the porridge (oatmeal).

Place the quinoa flakes, goji berries, cinnamon stick, 250ml (8fl oz/1 cup) of the macadamia nut milk and 475ml (16fl oz/scant 2 cups) of the water in a pan. Stir continuously over a medium heat for 2–3 minutes, then crush the raspberries into the pan, add the remaining water and stir for another 2 minutes, until piping hot.

Heat the remaining macadamia milk in a separate pan.

Spoon the porridge (oatmeal) into 4 bowls, pour over the hot macadamia milk and serve sprinkled with the pomegranate seeds.

Macadamia Nut Milk

200g (7oz/1⅓ cups) raw macadamia nuts, soaked for about 4 hours and drained
750ml–1 litre (1¼–1¾ pints/3–4 cups) purified or filtered water

Blend the ingredients in a Vitamix or high-speed blender until smooth, then filter through a muslin bag or a very fine strainer.

Store for up to 2 days in the fridge in a glass jar with an airtight lid.

Raw Buckwheat and Cinnamon Granola

Buckwheat is a great source of rutin, helping to strengthen the capillaries and veins throughout the body, supporting the cardiovascular system and helping to prevent thread and varicose veins in the legs.

Soak the buckwheat overnight in cold water, then rinse well (the discarded soaking water will be slimy and gelatinous), cover with fresh water and leave to soak and plump up for another day. Rinse again and drain well. Alternatively, bring the buckwheat to the boil, then simmer over a low heat for 15 minutes. Rinse in cold water, drain well and proceed with the recipe as follows.

Place all the ingredients in a bowl and mix well, then spread them in a thin layer on a dehydrator sheet and place in the dehydrator at 40–43°C/105–110°F for 10 hours.

Alternatively, spread the mixture in a thin layer on a baking tray (cookie sheet) and either place in the oven at the lowest temperature with the door open (or in the warming oven of an Aga) for 10 hours, or bake in a preheated oven at 110°C/225°F/gas mark ¼ for 1 hour.

Let the mixture cool completely before serving with yogurt or dairy-free milk and fresh fruit.

serves 2

♥♥♥⊤

150g (5oz/generous ¾ cup) raw buckwheat groats

75g (3oz/½ cup) raw almonds, soaked overnight and drained

75g (3oz/½ cup) mixed raw pumpkin, sunflower and flax seeds

1 tsp cinnamon

75g (3oz/scant ½ cup) mixed raisins and chopped dried figs

3 tbsp agave syrup

1 tbsp desiccated coconut (dry unsweetened shredded coconut)

To serve

Yogurt or a dairy-free milk (see pages 53 and 57)

Fresh fruit of your choice

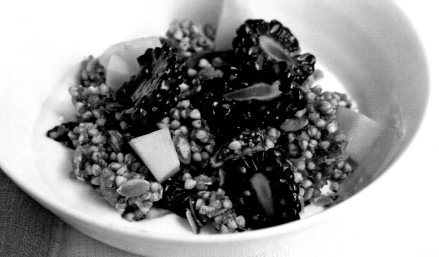

NUTRITIONAL NUGGET

Cinnamon is a potent anti-inflammatory, helping to settle bloating, wind and general abdominal discomfort.

Nut and Berry Layered Breakfast

serves 2–4

♥ ♥ ⍦

100g (3½oz/1 cup) raw walnuts

100g (3½oz/scant ⅔ cup) raw almonds

50g (2oz/⅓ cup) raw pumpkin seeds

50g (2oz/scant ⅓ cup) raw sunflower seeds

50g (2oz/⅓ cup) raw flax seeds

1 large punnet of blueberries

1 large punnet of raspberries

1 quantity of Raw Vanilla Cashew Cream (see below)

Keep your larder well stocked with nuts and seeds so you can throw this yummy breakfast together in minutes (remember to allow time for soaking).

Soak all the nuts and seeds for 30 minutes to 1 hour and drain. Then tip them into a food processor and pulse briefly – just enough to coarsely chop, but still retain their wonderful crunchy texture.

To serve, place a layer of berries in the bottom of a glass, place a layer of nut mix on top, and spoon over a layer of the Raw Vanilla Cashew Cream. Repeat the layers and decorate with berries. Repeat to make the number of servings you require.

Raw Vanilla Cashew Cream

♥ ♥ ⍦

100g (3½oz/⅔ cup) raw cashews, soaked for 1 hour and drained

60–125ml (2½–4fl oz/¼–½ cup) purified or filtered water

1 tsp vanilla extract

Drain the nuts and put in a blender. Add 60ml (2½fl oz/¼ cup) of the water and blend, adding more water as necessary to make a smooth cream, then add the vanilla extract and blend for a few more seconds.

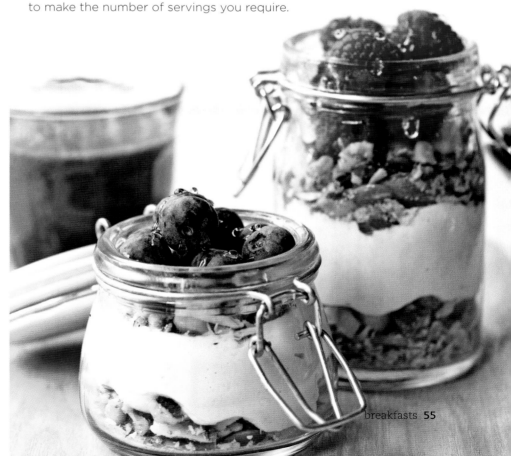

Nutty Granola

serves 4

50g (2oz/generous ¼ cup) dried
   dates
100g (3½oz/generous 1 cup)
   jumbo rolled oats
2 tbsp honey
85g (3¼oz/½ cup) mixed raw
   cashews and pecans
15g (½oz/1¾ tbsp) raw
   pumpkin seeds
3 tbsp olive oil

This is simply amazing. Make a batch and store in an airtight glass container and use it as a breakfast cereal or a crunchy topping on yogurt or porridge (oatmeal).

Preheat the oven to 160°C/325°F/gas mark 3.

Simmer the dates in 1cm (½in) water until soft and then blend until smooth. Stir in the remaining ingredients and mix well.

Spread the mixture on a baking tray (cookie sheet) and bake for 15 minutes until golden, then reduce the oven temperature to 110°C/225°F/gas mark ¼ and bake for a further 30 minutes or until the mixture is dry and crisp.

Leave to cool completely, then store in an airtight container.

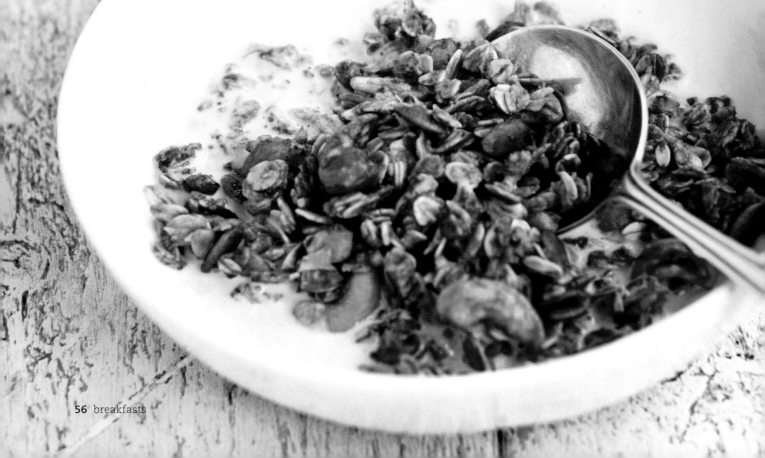

Milks

These milks are well worth the planning, although they don't take that much effort to make. They are all excellent alternatives to dairy milk.

Almond Milk

150g (5oz/scant 1 cup) raw almonds, soaked for 4 hours and drained
750ml–1 litre (1¼–1¾ pints/3–4 cups) purified or filtered water

Hemp Milk

150g (5oz/scant 1¼ cups) shelled hemp seeds, soaked for 4 hours and drained
1.2 litres (2 pints/5 cups) purified or filtered water

Brazil Nut Milk

125g (4oz/¾ cup) raw Brazil nuts, soaked for 4 hours and drained
750ml–1 litre (1¼–1¾ pints/3–4 cups) purified or filtered water

Brown Rice Milk

125g (4oz/¾ cup) cooked brown rice, soaked for 4 hours before cooking
475ml (16fl oz/scant 2 cups) purified or filtered water

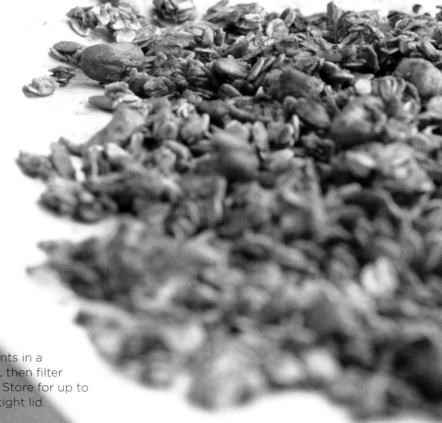

To make any milk, simply blend the ingredients in a Vitamix or high-speed blender until smooth, then filter through a muslin bag or a very fine strainer. Store for up to 2 days in the fridge in a glass jar with an airtight lid.

The Full HH Breakfast

serves 2

6 asparagus spears, trimmed

1 stem of vine-ripened baby
   tomatoes, divided into 2

2 portobello mushrooms, sliced

1 small garlic clove, sliced

1½ tsp olive oil

30g (1¼oz) goat's Cheddar,
   grated

4 eggs

200g (7oz) spinach

Juice of ½ lemon

Freshly ground black pepper

Gluten/wheat-free bread, to
   serve (optional)

NUTRITIONAL NUGGET
Eggs are a source of the essential
nutrient choline – vital for a
healthy brain and smart thinking.

Who said a full English need be greasy and fattening? Not in our book! Perfect for a Sunday brunch or even a scruffy supper. You can play with the recipe – scramble or boil the eggs, and add whatever is in the fridge.

Preheat the oven to 180°C/350°F/gas mark 4.

Place the asparagus, tomatoes on their vines and the mushrooms with garlic on top on a baking tray (cookie sheet), drizzle with a teaspoon of the olive oil and bake for 20 minutes (cherry tomatoes work well, too, but they'll need a bit less time, just till the skins split).

Remove from the oven and sprinkle the grated goat's cheese on the mushrooms and allow to melt.

Meanwhile, fill a frying pan with water to within 2.5cm (1in) of the top, bring to the boil, then reduce the heat to a simmer. When the asparagus and mushrooms have been in the oven for 15 minutes, crack the eggs very carefully into the simmering water and poach for 3 minutes, making sure that the water completely covers the eggs – if necessary, spoon the cooking water over the eggs while they cook.

Place the spinach in a bowl, cover with boiling water and leave to stand for 2 minutes, then drain well and add the remaining olive oil and the lemon juice. Divide between 2 serving plates.

Carefully remove the eggs from the water with a slotted spoon and arrange on the spinach. Place some mushroom on each plate with the asparagus and the vine tomatoes. Sprinkle with black pepper.

Serve immediately, with a piece of gluten-/wheat-free bread, if liked.

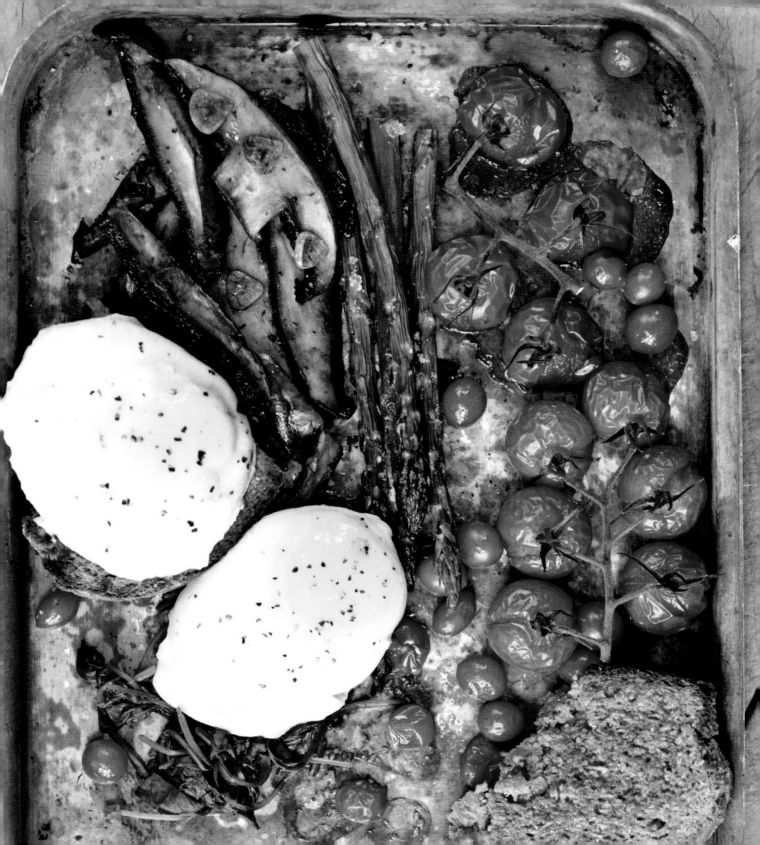

Scrambled Eggs and Baked Portobello Mushroom with Melted Goat's Cheese

serves 1

1 large portobello mushroom

1 tbsp olive oil

Pinch of Himalayan pink salt

20g (¾oz) firm goat's cheese, sliced

2 eggs

1 egg yolk

2 tbsp finely chopped dill, plus extra for garnishing (optional)

NUTRITIONAL NUGGET

All mushrooms are a fantastic source of vitamin D, which most of us lack if we are not living in sunny climates – so stock up in the winter on this sunshine food.

Scrambling eggs takes only minutes – but, remember, to make them oh-so-creamy cook over a low, low heat and stir constantly. By adding different herb combinations, you can make this dish your own.

Preheat the oven to 170°C/340°F/gas mark 3½.

Place the mushroom on a baking tray (cookie sheet), drizzle with the olive oil and sprinkle with a pinch of salt. Bake for 15 minutes, then arrange the goat's cheese slices on top and return to the oven for 3 minutes to melt the cheese.

Beat the whole eggs and egg yolk in a bowl and add the dill, then pour them into a hot pan and cook over a low heat, stirring constantly, to the consistency you require.

Serve immediately with the mushroom and goat's cheese, with a little extra chopped dill if you like.

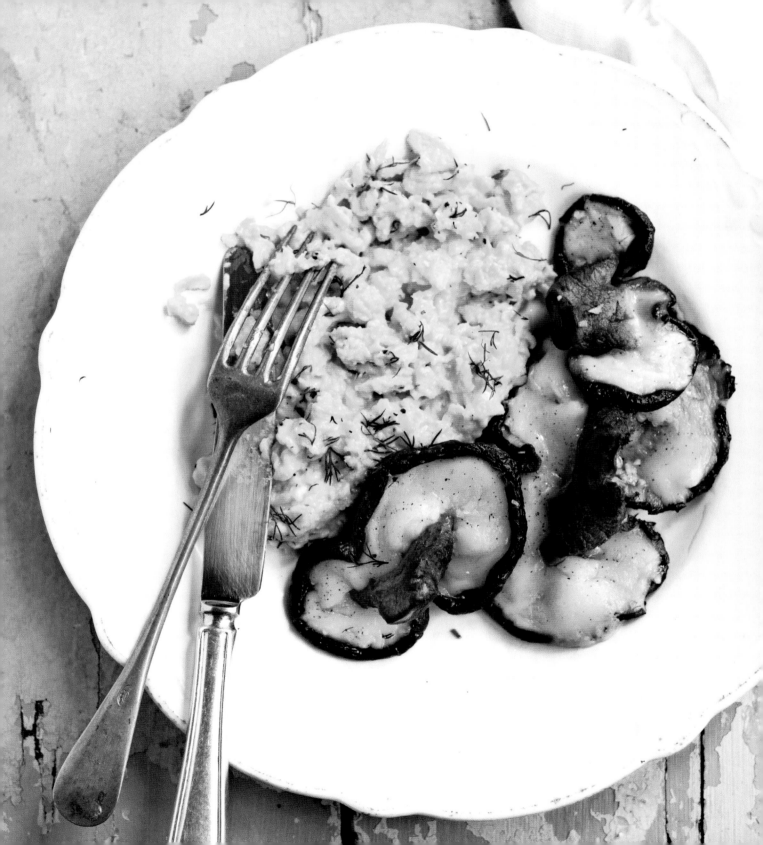

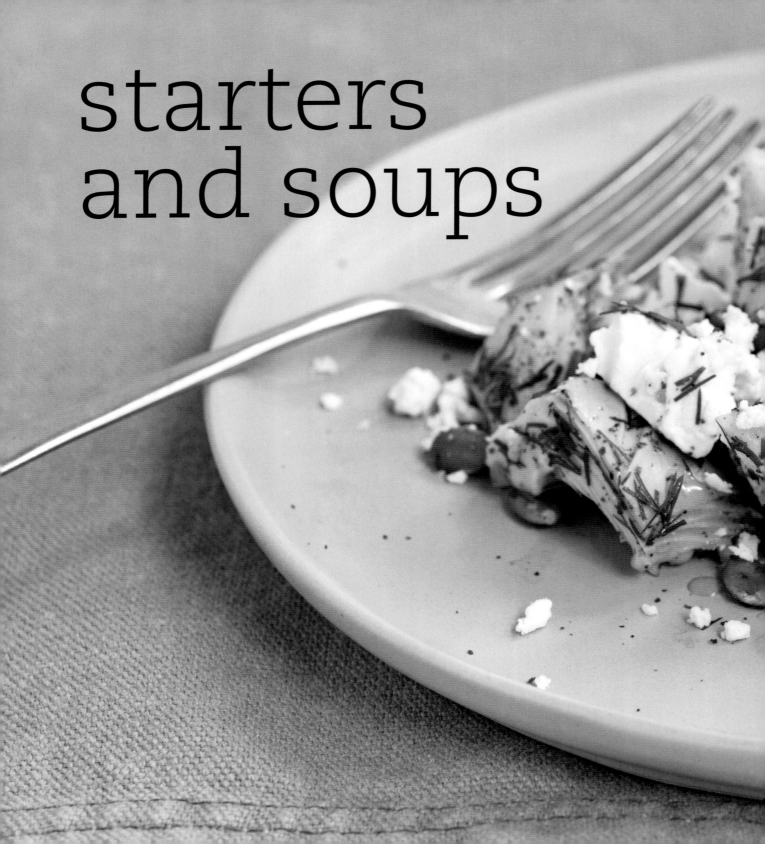

starters
and soups

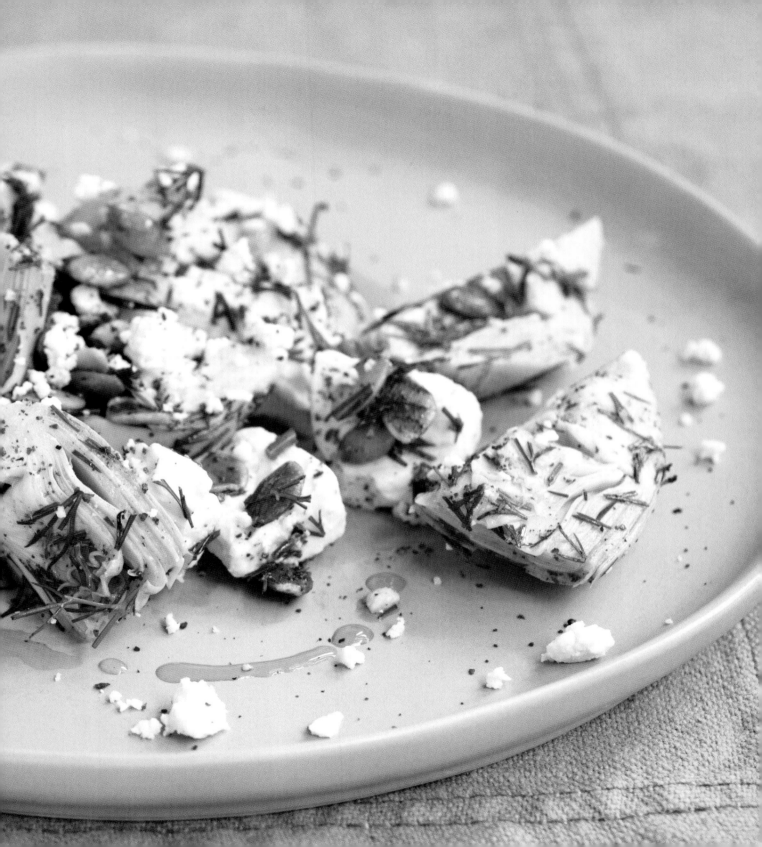

Artichoke Hearts with Feta

serves 2

200g (7oz) canned artichoke
    hearts, chopped
2 tsp extra virgin olive oil
Juice of 1 lemon
60g (2½oz) feta, diced
2 tbsp raw pumpkin seeds

To serve
Pinch of sumac
2 tbsp finely chopped dill

(Pictured on pages 62–63) This takes moments to prepare.
We've used canned artichoke hearts but you could try
roasted Jerusalem artichokes for a different flavour.

Mix the artichoke hearts with the olive oil and lemon juice in a bowl,
then gently fold in the feta and pumpkin seeds.

Serve garnished with sumac and chopped dill.

Cashew Dipping Sauce for Raw Summer Spring Rolls

75g (3oz/½ cup) raw cashews,
    soaked and drained
50g (2oz) cucumber, peeled and
    chopped
½ small red pepper, deseeded
    and chopped
1 small garlic clove
2 red chillies, deseeded
Dash or two of tamari sauce,
    to taste
Squeeze of lime juice
Squeeze of agave syrup

Place all the ingredients in a blender
and process briefly, then add water
a little at a time, processing after
each addition to make a smooth and
creamy sauce.

Transfer to a small bowl and serve
as a dipping sauce.

NUTRITIONAL NUGGET
Cashew nuts are a fantastic
source of niacin – a B
vitamin known to elevate
mood! A handful of cashews
is a natural alternative to
Prozac.

Raw Summer Spring Rolls

serves 2

4 rice paper rounds

1 nori seaweed sheet, cut into
　4 squares

1 carrot, cut into julienne strips

1 courgette (zucchini), cut into
　julienne strips

1 spring onion (scallion), cut
　into fine strips

1 small cucumber, cut into
　julienne strips

Chunk of Chinese leaf lettuce,
　shredded

1 packet beansprouts

1 handful of coriander
　(cilantro), chopped

100g (3½oz) smoked tofu, diced

Practice makes perfect with these little parcels. At first it's a little fiddly but you'll get the hang of it in no time. The trick here is not to over-soak the rice paper rounds.

Soak the rice paper rounds in cold water for about 1 minute to just soften them, then remove from the water and pat dry. Lay each rice paper round on a flat surface and place a nori square on top of each.

Arrange a medley of vegetables, tofu and coriander (cilantro) in the centre of each paper/nori wrapper. Roll the edge nearest to you over the filling and then tuck in the outside edges. Continue to roll carefully but tightly. This does take a little practice, but delicate handling will get you there in a short time.

Serve alongside the Cashew Dipping Sauce (see opposite) and perhaps some watercress or salad leaves (salad greens).

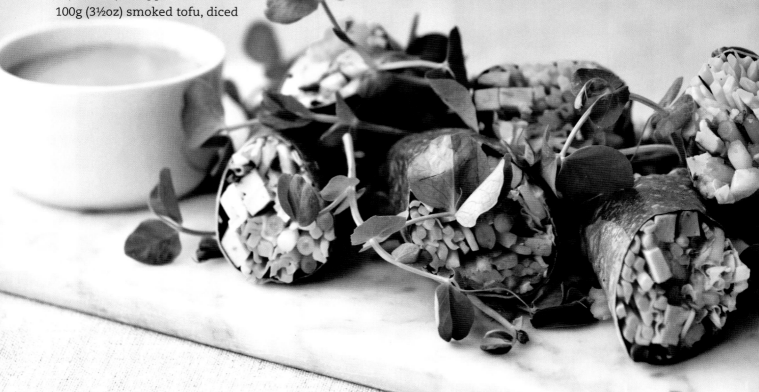

Stuffed Round Courgettes

serves 2

2 small round courgettes
   (zucchini)
1 tsp olive oil
3 garlic cloves
1 small onion, finely chopped
50g (2oz) carrot, finely grated
1 tsp thyme leaves
1 tsp oregano leaves
2 canned artichoke hearts,
   chopped
½ tsp grated lemon zest
½ tsp Himalayan pink salt
20g (¾oz/scant ¼ cup) raw
   cashews, chopped
25g (1 oz) feta, crumbled

To serve
Rocket (arugula) leaves
Cherry tomatoes
Radish sprouts
Extra virgin olive oil,
   for drizzling

Beautiful to present on the table for a dinner party as a starter or even as your main course, served with brown rice and a crunchy salad. If you are vegan, just leave out the feta as the cashews provide plenty of protein.

Preheat the oven to 150°C/300°F/gas mark 2. Next, trim the stalks off the courgettes (zucchini). Brush a roasting tin with ½ teaspoon of the olive oil, add the courgettes (zucchini) and garlic and roast for 50 minutes, until tender. Remove from the oven, leaving the oven on. When the courgettes (zucchini) are cool enough to handle, carefully scoop out the flesh and set aside.

Heat the remaining oil in a pan and gently sauté the onion for 5 minutes. Add the carrot, thyme and oregano and sauté for a further 5 minutes, or until the carrot is soft. Add the courgette (zucchini) flesh and chopped artichoke hearts and sauté for 2 minutes.

Stir in the lemon zest, salt and chopped cashews. Divide the mixture between the courgette (zucchini) shells, stuffing it in tightly. Top with the crumbled feta and return to the oven for 15–20 minutes or until the feta is golden.

Serve the courgettes (zucchini) with the Fig Jam (see below) and a simple salad of rocket (arugula) leaves, cherry tomatoes and peppery radish sprouts, drizzled with a good olive oil.

Fig Jam

100g (3½oz) figs
2 tsp balsamic vinegar
1 tsp rice syrup
1 tbsp water

While the courgettes (zucchini) are in the oven, chop the figs and place in a saucepan with the balsamic vinegar, rice syrup and water. Simmer gently until the figs become soft and sticky.

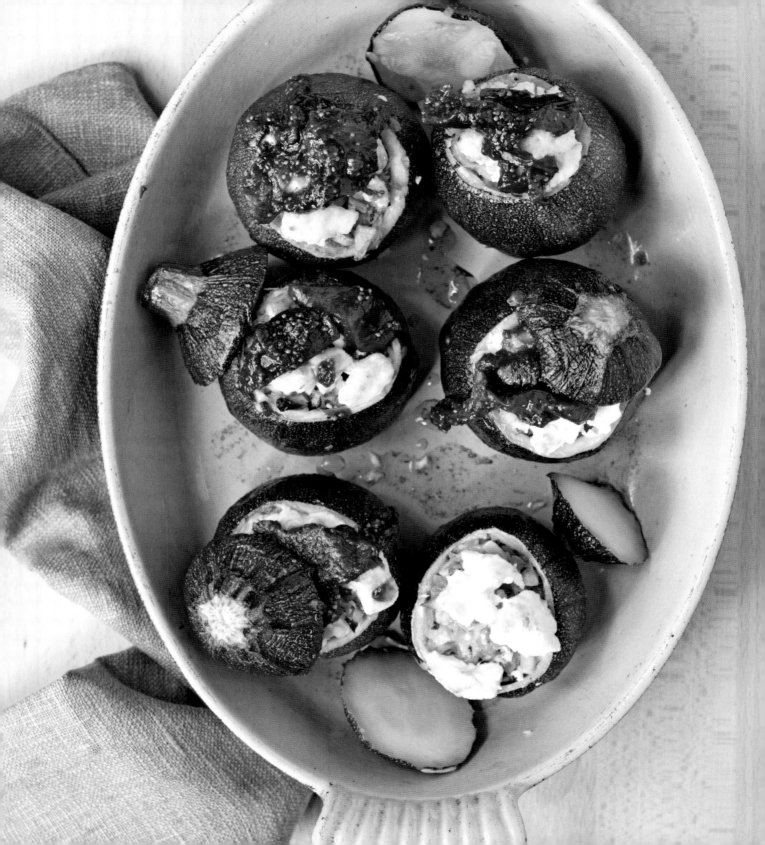

Pak Choi Parcels

makes 6

2 tsp toasted sesame oil

85g (3¼oz) aubergine (eggplant), cut into julienne strips

2 garlic cloves, minced

1 tbsp water

70g (2¾oz) carrot, grated

45g (1¾oz) water chestnuts, cut into julienne strips

15g (½oz/1¾ tbsp) mixed raw black and white sesame seeds, toasted

½ tsp tamari

1 tsp white miso paste

20g (¾oz) dried sliced mushrooms, soaked in hot water until softened

6 outer pak choi leaves

Sprouts, to garnish

These beautiful parcels are totally divine. A little bit fiddly to construct, but once you bite into them they just explode with flavour in your mouth.

First, make the Black Bean Sauce (see below). To make the filling for the parcels, heat a frying pan and add the sesame oil. Add the aubergine (eggplant) and garlic and sauté for 2 minutes. Stir in the water, then add the carrot and water chestnuts and stir-steam ('fry' with water to create steam to sweat the vegetables) for a further 5 minutes, until softened. Mix in the sesame seeds and tamari, then transfer the filling to a bowl and set aside.

Return the pan to the heat and add the miso paste and a splash of water. Spread the miso around the pan to heat through, then return the filling to the pan with the mushrooms and stir well.

To assemble the parcels, steam the pak choi leaves for 3–5 minutes, until just tender. Trim off the stalks, leaving a little to keep the leaf intact. Place the leaf on a board with the stem end facing you. Place a spoonful of the filling in the centre of the leaf at the stem end, then roll the stem end over the filling, fold in the sides and very carefully roll up the parcel so the filling is securely enclosed.

Serve immediately with the Black Bean Sauce or refrigerate and steam for 2 minutes just before serving and garnish with sprouts.

Black Bean Sauce

1 tsp light sesame oil

100g (3½oz/scant ⅔ cup) Chinese fermented black beans

1 garlic clove, minced

2 tsp grated fresh root ginger

½ tsp oregano

½ tsp ground cumin

¼ tsp grated orange zest

100ml (3½fl oz/generous ⅓ cup) water

1 tbsp rice vinegar

½ tbsp tamari

1 tsp agave syrup

To make the sauce, heat the sesame oil in a pan over a medium-high heat. Add the beans and garlic and stir for 1 minute, then add the remaining ingredients and stir until the sauce thickens.

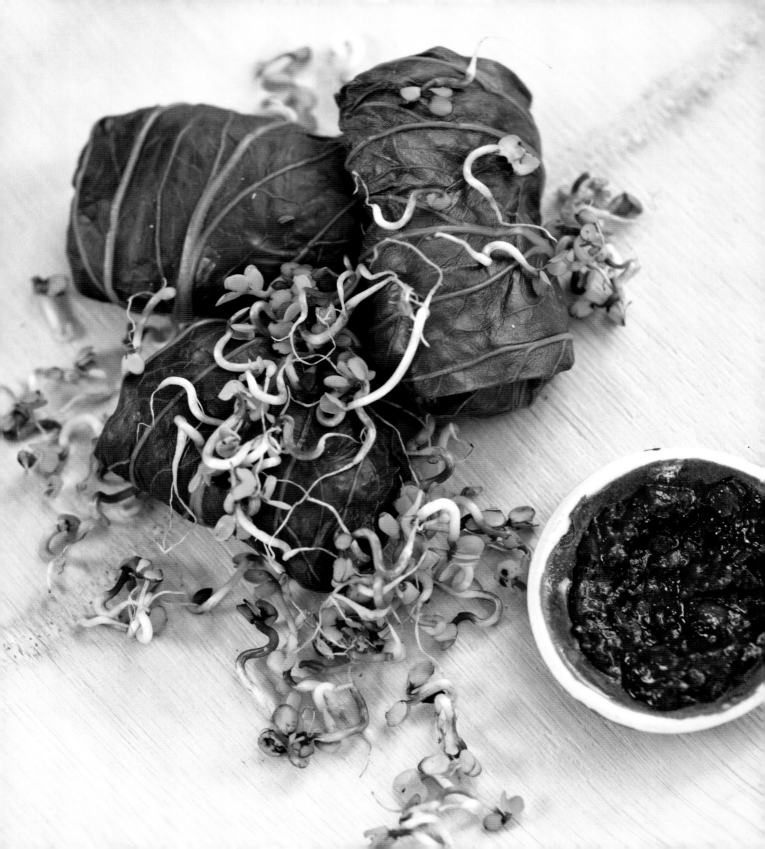

Falafel Wraps

serves 2

50g (2oz/scant ½ cup) ground raw flax seeds

50g (2oz/⅓ cup) raw sesame seeds

2 carrots, peeled and thinly sliced

2 portobello mushrooms, cut into small dice

½ small onion, finely chopped

1 garlic clove, finely chopped

3 tbsp olive oil

Pinch of Himalayan pink salt

150g (5oz/1 cup) pistachios

125g (4oz/generous ¾ cup) raw almonds

150g (5oz/scant 1 cup) raw sunflower seeds, soaked for 30 minutes and drained

1 tbsp finely chopped parsley

¾ tsp ground cumin

1 tsp lemon juice

Freshly ground black pepper

To serve (see opposite)
Iceberg Lettuce Wraps
Mint Yogurt
Tomato Salsa

Cooking a variety of seeds, like this, at a very low temperature in the oven protects the essential fats that they provide and ensures that the flavour remains fresh and the taste crunchy.

Preheat the oven to 110°C/225°F/gas mark ¼.

Combine the ground flax seeds and sesame seeds in a bowl and set aside.

Combine the carrots, mushrooms, onion, garlic and 2 tablespoons of the olive oil in a separate bowl. Add a pinch of salt and mix well. Place the pistachios, almonds and sunflower seeds in a food processor and process to a crumbly texture. Add the nut mixture to the vegetable mixture, together with the parsley, cumin and lemon juice. Mix thoroughly and season to taste with black pepper.

Form the mixture into balls 3–4cm (1¼–1¾in) in diameter. Roll the falafel balls in the flax- and sesame-seed mix to coat well. Place on a baking tray (cookie sheet) and bake for about 40 minutes, or until crisp on the outside but still moist.

Serve the falafels, lettuce wraps, tomato salsa and mint yogurt in separate bowls. To assemble, place 3 falafels in a lettuce wrap and add a spoonful each of tomato salsa and mint yogurt.

For the Iceburg Lettuce Wraps
1 iceberg lettuce

Chop the root off the lettuce and carefully peel away the large outer leaves. Place them in a large bowl of cold water until you are ready to serve, to keep them crisp and fresh. Pat dry to use.

Mint Yogurt

250g (8oz/scant 1 cup) soya yogurt
25g (1oz) mint leaves

Place the yogurt in a bowl. Just before serving, finely chop the mint and stir into the yogurt (don't chop before you are ready as the mint will turn black).

Tomato Salsa

400g (13oz) tomatoes, finely diced
75g (3oz) red onion, finely diced
1 small cucumber, deseeded and finely diced
1 red chilli, deseeded and finely diced
½ garlic clove, grated
2 tbsp olive oil
Juice of 1 lime

Place all the ingredients in a bowl and mix gently to combine.

Stuffed New Potatoes

makes 10/serves 2

5 new potatoes
2 tbsp olive oil, plus extra for brushing
Pinch of Himalayan pink salt
Pinch of ground cumin
125g (4oz) canned artichoke hearts
100g (3½oz/½ cup) cooked cannellini beans
Juice of 1 lemon
1 tsp sumac, plus extra to garnish

Preheat the oven to 170°C/340°F/gas mark 3½.

Put the potatoes in an ovenproof dish, brush with olive oil and sprinkle with the salt. Bake for 45 minutes, or until tender. Remove from the oven and leave to cool for 15 minutes, leaving the oven on.

When the potatoes are cool enough to handle, cut each one in half and carefully scoop out and discard the flesh (this can be mashed or used in soup). Place the scooped-out skins on a baking tray (cookie sheet), sprinkle with cumin, then return to the oven for a further 15 minutes until crisp and golden. Set aside to cool.

To make the dip, process the remaining ingredients in a blender.

Serve the potato skins filled with the bean dip, garnished with a sprinkle of sumac.

Patty Pan Squash Canapés

makes 8/serves 2

6 dried porcini mushrooms
8 patty pan squash (baby yellow squash)
1 tbsp olive oil
1 garlic clove, diced
100g (3½oz) curly kale (thick stems removed), roughly chopped
3 tbsp finely chopped parsley
1 large beef tomato, deseeded and finely diced
1 tbsp soft goat's cheese

Soak the mushrooms in hot water for 30 minutes, drain on kitchen paper for 2 minutes, then dice.

Preheat the oven to 170°C/340°F/gas mark 3½. Place the patty pan squash (baby yellow squash) on a baking tray (cookie sheet) and bake for 20 minutes, or until the skins are soft and slightly wrinkled. Remove and set aside to cool.

Meanwhile, heat the olive oil in a pan over a low heat and gently sauté the garlic for 1 minute. Add the diced soaked mushroom, kale and parsley and stir continuously for a further 1 minute. Add the diced tomato and stir for a further 2 minutes, then remove from the heat.

When the squash are cool enough to handle, cut off the tops with a small knife and carefully scoop out the flesh with a teaspoon, leaving a 5mm (¼in) shell and keeping the skin intact.

Just before serving, add the goat's cheese to the mushroom, kale and tomato mixture, and heat through to melt the cheese. Stuff the patty pan squash with the filling and serve warm.

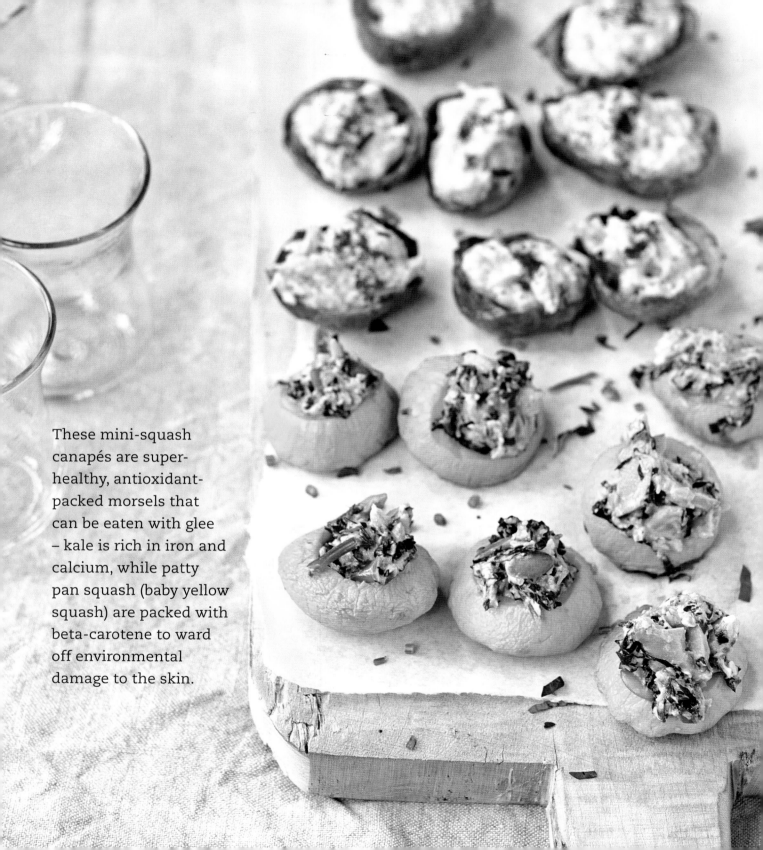

These mini-squash canapés are super-healthy, antioxidant-packed morsels that can be eaten with glee – kale is rich in iron and calcium, while patty pan squash (baby yellow squash) are packed with beta-carotene to ward off environmental damage to the skin.

Aubergine and Pesto Rolls

makes 6 rolls/serves 2

125g (4oz) aubergine (eggplant)

3 tbsp olive oil

30g (1¼oz/scant ¼ cup) pine nuts

5g (¼oz) flat-leaf parsley

1 small garlic clove

20g (¾oz) feta, crumbled

25g (1oz) rocket (arugula) leaves

These little beauties are so delicious and versatile. You could serve these starters on a platter at a party or team with a vibrant salad for a simple supper for two.

Preheat the oven to 170°C/340°F/gas mark 3½.

Slice the aubergine (eggplant) lengthways into 6 x 5mm (¼in) slices. Place on a baking tray (cookie sheet) lined with greaseproof paper, drizzle with 1 tablespoon of the olive oil and bake in the oven for 15 minutes, or until tender. Set aside to cool.

Meanwhile, whizz the pine nuts, parsley, garlic and remaining olive oil to a rough paste in a blender.

Divide the pesto between the aubergine (eggplant) slices and spread it down the centre. Top each one with the feta, roll up the aubergine (eggplant) slices and secure with cocktail sticks (toothpicks).

To serve, arrange the rocket (arugula) on 2 plates and top with 3 rolls.

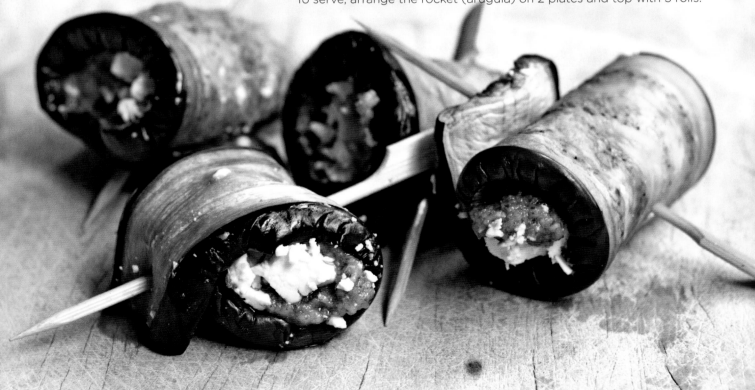

Dill Steamed Artichokes

You cannot beat the satisfaction of eating a globe artichoke – it's a meal in itself – or serve it as a starter (appetiser) for a dinner party.

serves 1

1 artichoke
1 tbsp olive oil
1 garlic clove
3 tbsp finely chopped dill
225ml (7½fl oz/scant 1 cup)
   purifed or filtered water

For the dressing
2 tbsp tamari
1 tbsp balsamic vinegar
2 tbsp olive oil
1 tbsp agave syrup

Chop the long stem off the artichoke, leaving just a short one.

Heat the olive oil in a very deep pan, then gently sauté the garlic for 1 minute. Stir in 2 tablespoons of the chopped dill.

Add the water and then the artichoke, stem pointing upwards. Cover the pan and steam over a low heat for 45–55 minutes, topping up with water when necessary. The artichoke is cooked when you can pull the leaves out easily and the 'flesh' is tender.

Meanwhile, whisk together all the dressing ingredients.

Serve the artichoke sprinkled with the remaining chopped dill and accompanied with the dressing in a pot on the side.

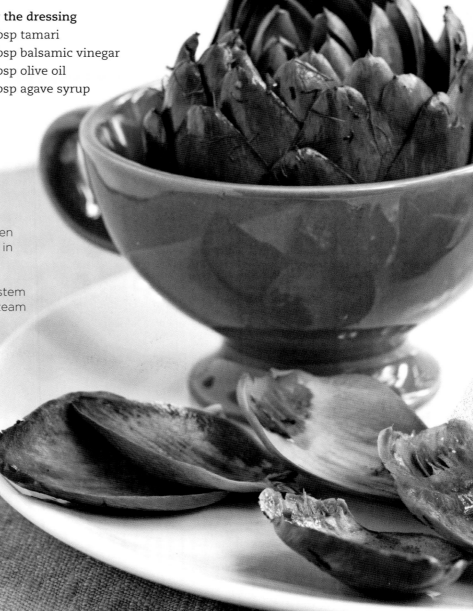

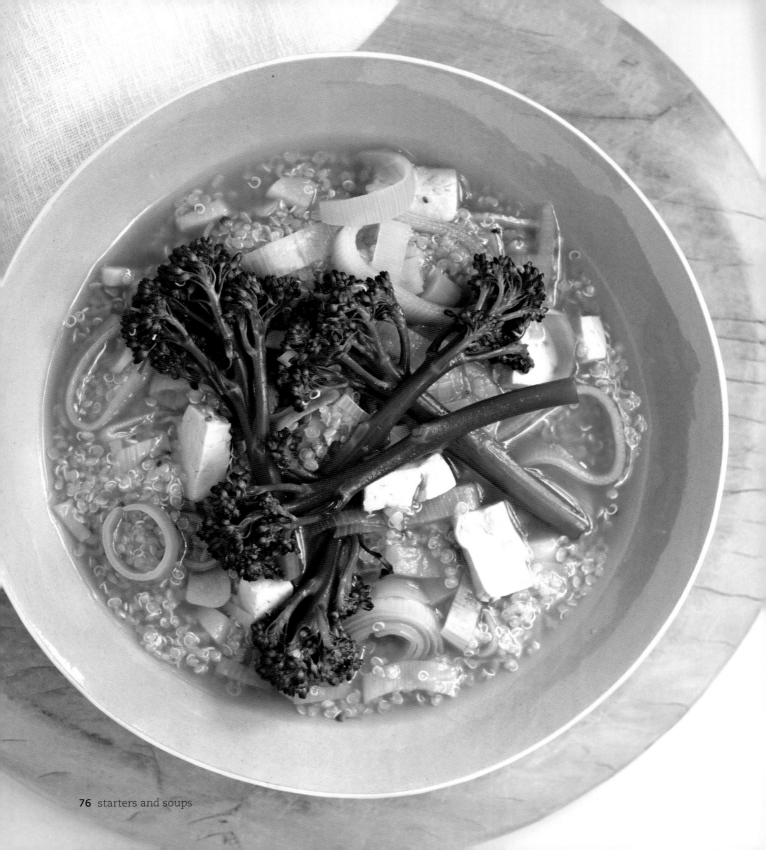

Do as the Chinese do, 'warm your body's cooker' by starting your meal with a soup. If you want to eat mainly raw in the winter, make sure you have either a small bowl of soup or a glass of hot water prior to your raw meal, as this helps to digest your food more effectively.

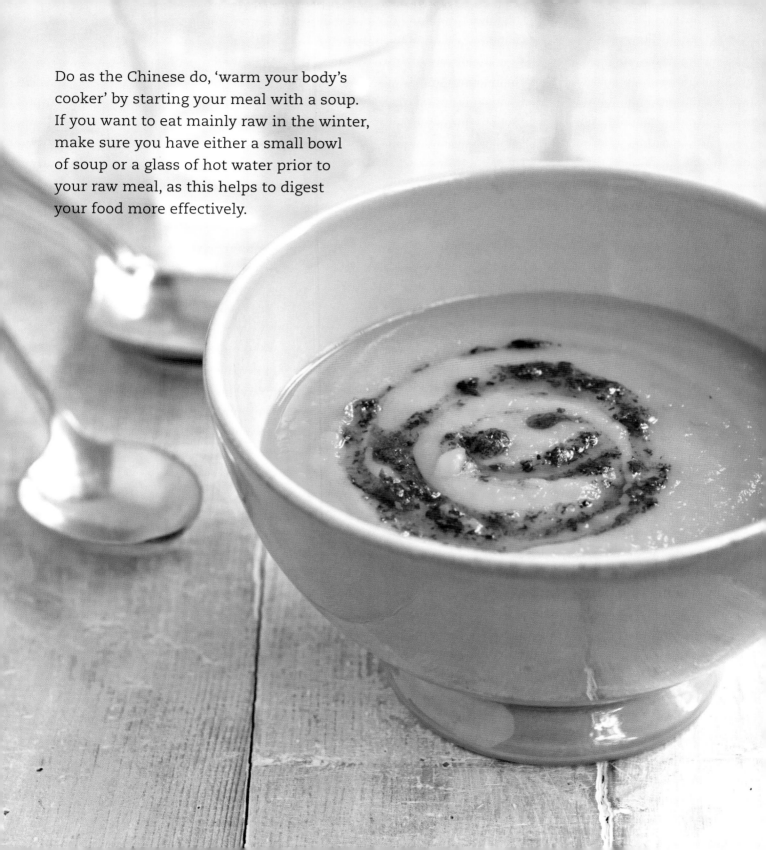

Vegetable and Quinoa Warming Soup

serves 2

60g (2½oz/⅓ cup) quinoa

1½ tsp bouillon powder

225ml (7½fl oz/scant 1 cup)
   purified or filtered water

6 tenderstem broccoli stalks,
   chopped

100g (3½oz) leeks, chopped

Juice of 2 limes

2 tsp tamari

80g (3oz) tofu, cut into cubes

4 tbsp finely chopped coriander
   (cilantro), to garnish
   (optional)

(Pictured on page 76.) This gentle, warming soup is a great addition to your repertoire. You can add whatever vegetables you have in your refrigerator – it's a staple request in my house on a Sunday night!

Measure the volume of the quinoa and bring twice the volume of water to the boil in a pan. Add the quinoa and the bouillon powder, bring back to the boil, then simmer for 5 minutes.

Boil the measured water and add to the pan with the broccoli and leeks, lime juice and tamari and simmer for a further 5 minutes.

Add the tofu and simmer for a further 2 minutes, until the tofu is heated through.

Serve garnished with chopped coriander (cilantro) if wished.

NUTRITIONAL NUGGET
Did you know that soaking your nuts and seeds at least 2 hours before eating re-activates the enzymes making them a 'live' food, that is easier to digest making your snack, meal or juice super-nutritious.

Butternut Squash Soup

serves 4

3 tbsp olive oil

1 red onion, chopped

1 large garlic clove, chopped

600ml (1 pint/2½ cups) purified
   or filtered water

750g (1½lb) butternut squash,
   peeled weight, deseeded and
   chopped

1 large carrot, chopped

1 tsp bouillon powder

1 red chilli, deseeded and
   chopped

½ tsp finely grated fresh
   root ginger

1 tsp lemon juice

**For the coriander (cilantro) and
   parsley oil**

Leaves from ½ small bunch of
   coriander (cilantro), finely
   chopped

Leaves from ½ small bunch
   of flat-leaf parsley, finely
   chopped

6 tbsp olive oil

Pinch of ground cumin

(Pictured on page 77.) I love making soups – they are so delicious. If you make batches and freeze them in portions, all you have to do is simply defrost and reheat – so you always have a tasty, nutritious meal to hand.

Heat the olive oil in a large pan, add the onion and garlic and sauté gently for 5 minutes until softened, then add 5 teaspoons of the water and continue cooking until the onion absorbs the water.

Add the butternut squash and carrot and cook gently until they start to sweat. Add the remaining water and the bouillon powder, bring to the boil and simmer for 15 minutes.

Next, pop the red chilli, ginger and lemon juice in the pan and simmer for a further 15 minutes.

Meanwhile, to make the herb oil, stir the chopped herbs into the oil with a pinch of cumin. Alternatively, whizz the whole leaves with the oil and cumin in a mini food processor until finely chopped.

Transfer the soup to a blender (or use a hand-held blender in the pan) and blend until smooth. Serve hot, drizzled with the coriander (cilantro) and parsley oil.

TIP

By simmering the ingredients over a low heat with splashes of water you start to layer the flavours, which really helps to bring out the subtle hits of each ingredient. The drizzle of herb oil is a perfect garnish.

Fennel and Pear Soup

serves 2

1 large fennel bulb, trimmed
1 tbsp olive oil, plus extra for
  drizzling
1 onion, sliced
1 garlic clove, chopped
600ml (1 pint/2½ cups)
  vegetable stock (made with
  ½ tsp bouillon powder)
1 pear, cored and chopped

NUTRITIONAL NUGGET
Fennel provides good support
to the liver for cleansing,
while both pear and fennel
are packed with potassium,
the most alkalising of all the
minerals. Potassium also helps
regulate fluid retention in the
body, ensuring that all nutrients
are delivered to where they are
needed, and preventing any
possibility of dehydration at a
cellular level.

This fabulous soup is one of my favourites. Both pear
and fennel are high in pectin, which help to draw
toxins out of the body, so this is a perfect candidate for
the Cleanse or Lifestyle phases. Its rich flavours and
creaminess are absolutely delicious and you just won't
believe that there is no naughtiness in it!

Slice the fennel bulb in half, then, using a very sharp knife, cut 4
thin slivers and set aside, covered, to use as a garnish. Chop the
remaining fennel.

Heat the olive oil in a large saucepan and sauté the onion and garlic,
adding 3 tablespoons of the stock when they start to dry out.

Add the chopped fennel, adding another 3 tablespoons of the
vegetable stock when this starts to dry out. Add the pear and the
remaining stock, bring to the boil, then simmer for 40 minutes, until
the fennel is wonderfully tender.

Transfer the vegetables and pear to a blender (or use a hand-held
blender in the pan) with some of the liquid and blend until smooth,
adding as much of the remaining liquid as necessary to make the
exact consistency you like.

Serve garnished with the reserved fennel and a swirl of olive oil.

WHAT IS BOUILLON POWDER?
Made only from vegetables, this stock powder gives
you instant stock whenever you need it or a touch of
saltiness if that's what's called for.

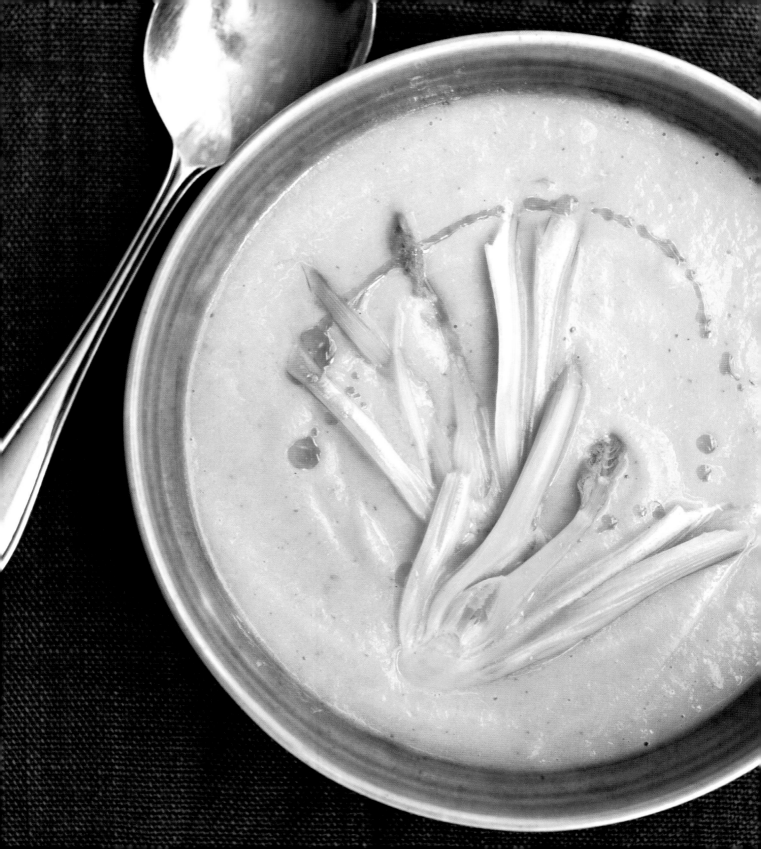

Mixed Vegetable and Soya Bean Hotpot

serves 4

2 tsp soya bean paste
900ml (1½ pints/3²⁄₃ cups)
    purified or filtered water
2 sprigs of lemon thyme
½ onion, cut into small dice
100g (3½oz) carrots, cut into
    large dice
100g (3½oz) potatoes, cut into
    large dice
100g (3½oz) pumpkin, cut into
    large dice
100g (3½oz) courgettes
    (zucchini), cut into large dice
100g (3½oz) mixed red and
    yellow peppers, deseeded
    and cut into large dice
100g (3½oz) firm tofu, cut into
    large dice

Simple, easy and clean is the motto for this little bowl of broth packed with vegetable goodness. It takes less than half an hour to make, perfect after a long day.

Dissolve the soya bean paste in the water in a large pan. Bring to the boil, add the lemon thyme sprigs, then simmer for 3-4 minutes to infuse the broth. Discard the lemon thyme sprigs.

Add the onion, carrots and potatoes and cook for 10 minutes. Add the pumpkin, courgettes (zucchini) and peppers and cook for a further 5-10 minutes, or until the vegetables are just tender.

Add the tofu and simmer for a further 2 minutes.

Serve immediately in warmed bowls and garnish with coriander and sliced spring onions (scallions) if wished.

NUTRITIONAL NUGGET
Tofu is a great source of vegetarian protein but we suggest you limit using soya products to three times a week as the phytoestrogens are potent.

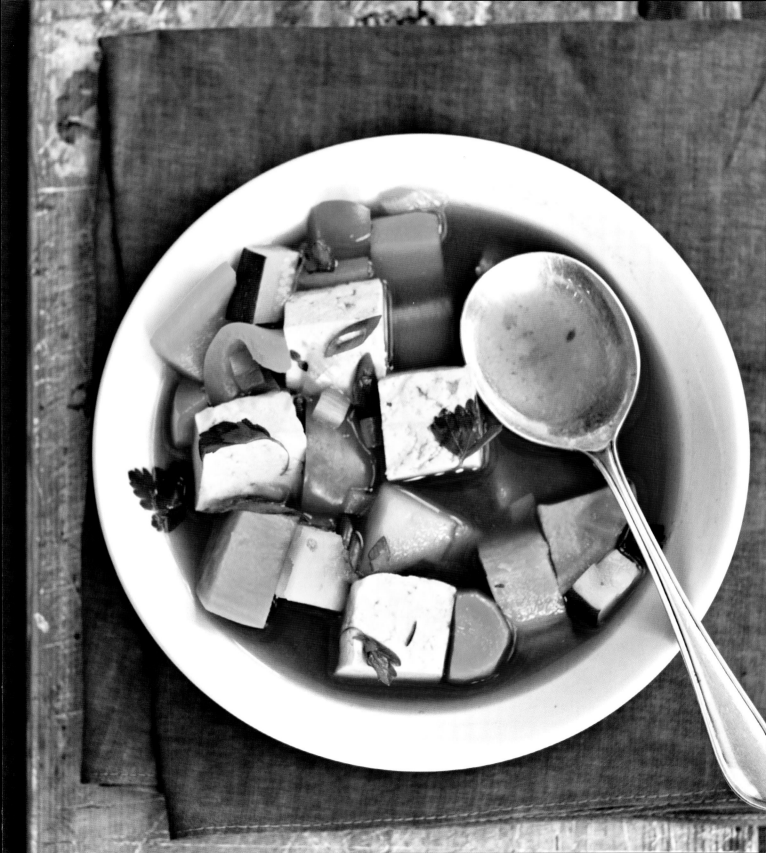

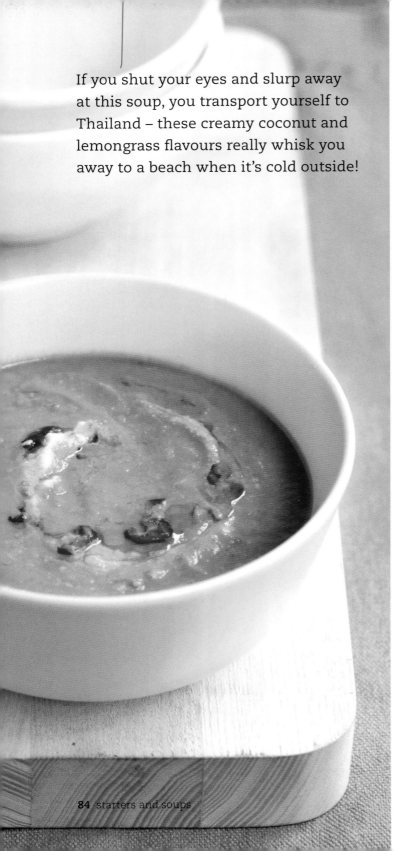

If you shut your eyes and slurp away at this soup, you transport yourself to Thailand – these creamy coconut and lemongrass flavours really whisk you away to a beach when it's cold outside!

Tomato, Coconut and Chilli Soup

serves 2

1 tbsp coconut oil
75g (3oz) shallots, chopped
20g (¾oz) fresh root ginger, chopped
1 garlic clove, chopped
½ red chilli, chopped
1 lemongrass stalk, chopped
1 tsp coriander seeds

300g (10oz) tomatoes, chopped
400ml (14fl oz/1⅔ cups) coconut milk
1 tsp tamari
1 tsp lime juice

To serve
Coconut cream
Chilli oil
Finely chopped coriander (cilantro) (optional)

Heat the coconut oil in a large pan. Add the shallots, ginger and garlic and sauté gently for 5 minutes, until softened. Add the chilli, lemongrass and coriander seeds and sauté for a further 5 minutes. Add the chopped tomatoes and sauté for a further 5 minutes.

Stir in the coconut milk, bring to the boil, then simmer for 30 minutes. Season with tamari and a little lime juice.

Transfer the soup to a blender (or use a hand-held blender in the pan) and blend until smooth. Pass through a fine sieve if you want it even smoother.

Serve hot, garnished with a swirl of coconut cream, a drizzle of chilli oil and, if you like, a sprinkle of chopped fresh coriander (cilantro).

White Gazpacho

This is a super-easy recipe. Almonds are the most alkaline of all nuts, and rich in magnesium to help you relax and sleep well. Add a swirl of olive oil to each bowl for added essential fats.

serves 4

400g (13oz/2 cups) canned cannellini beans

400g (13oz/2 cups) canned butter beans

150g (5oz/scant 1 cup) raw almonds

475ml (16fl oz/scant 2 cups) purified or filtered water

1 handful of mint

2 small cucumbers, peeled and chopped

225ml (7½fl oz/scant 1 cup) apple juice

1 tsp extra virgin olive oil, plus extra to garnish

Zest and juice of 1 lemon

1 red chilli, deseeded

1 handful of ice

First, rinse the canned beans and drain. Place the almonds, beans and water in a blender and blend until smooth, then add all the remaining ingredients, except the ice.

Just before serving, blend in the ice, then serve immediately, garnished with a swirl of olive oil and some strips of lemon zest, chilli and mint.

TIP

This is a variation on a classic Spanish soup that has been used for years to boost immunity and relieve digestive complaints.

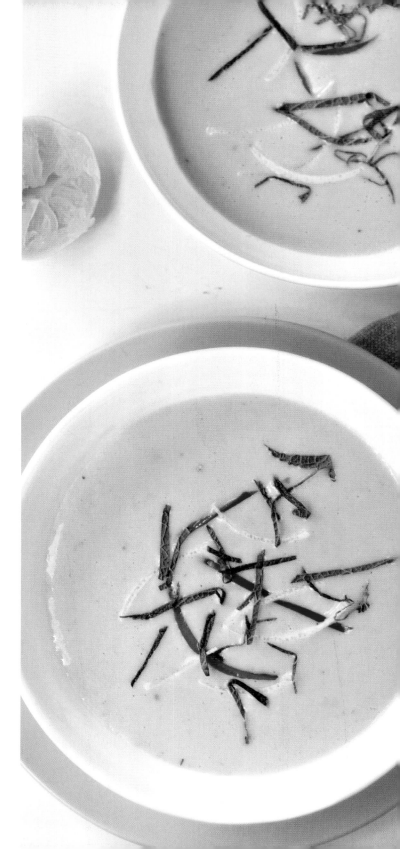

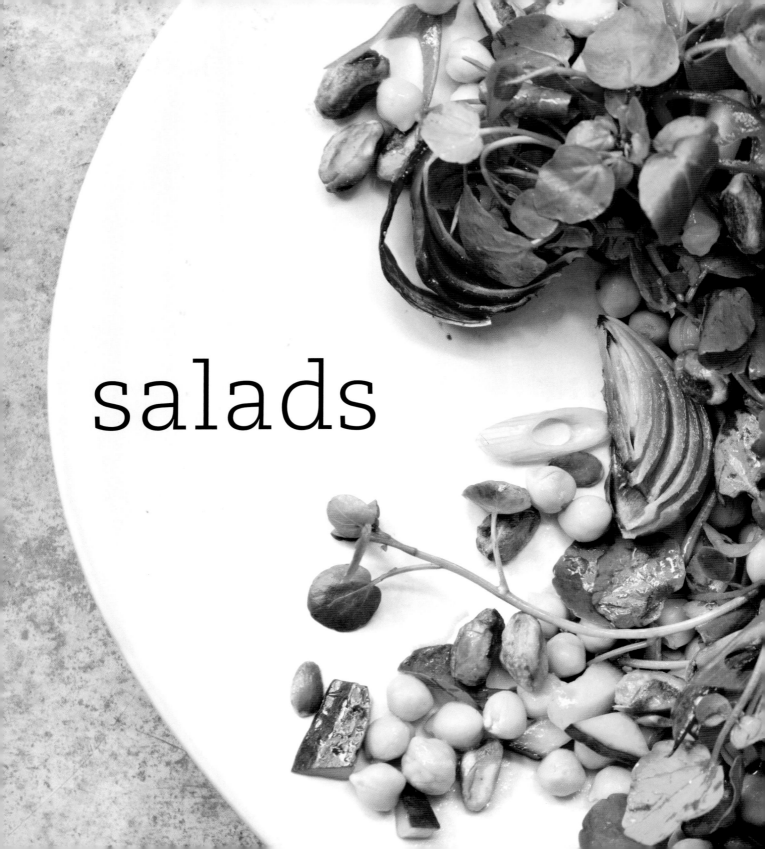

salads

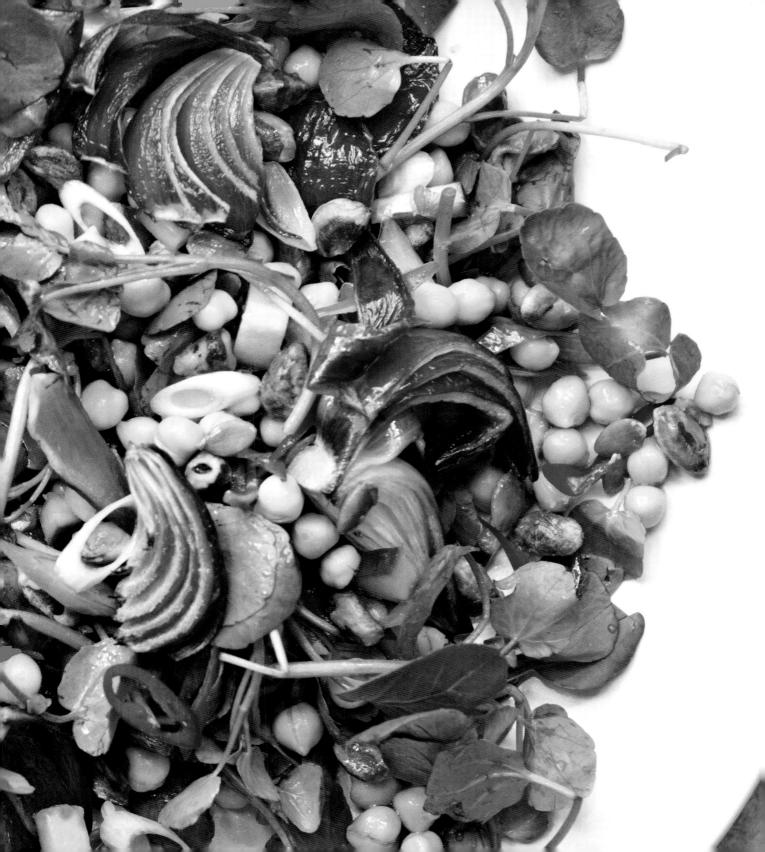

Watercress, Roasted Onion and Pistachio Salad

serves 1

½ red onion, cut into chunks

1 tbsp olive oil

30g (1¼oz/generous ⅛ cup) canned chickpeas, rinsed and drained

1 small garlic clove, finely grated

½ red chilli, finely sliced diagonally

15g (½oz) deseeded cucumber, finely sliced

15g (½oz) raw pumpkin seeds

15g (½oz) raw pistachios

70g (2¾oz) watercress

1 spring onion (scallion), sliced diagonally

For the dressing

2 tbsp olive oil

Juice of 1 lemon

1 tbsp tamari

1 tsp agave syrup

(Pictured on pages 86–87.) This salad is a show-stopper – I love to make a big platter, put it in the middle of the table and let people serve themselves, but it also makes a great supper for one if you are having a quiet night in.

Preheat the oven to 170°C/340°F/gas mark 3½.

Place the onion chunks on a baking tray (cookie sheet), drizzle with the olive oil and bake for 30 minutes, or until soft.

Place the chickpeas in a bowl with the roasted onion and the garlic and mix thoroughly. Stir in the chilli, cucumber, pumpkin seeds and pistachios.

Whisk the dressing ingredients together with a fork.

To serve, scatter the watercress on a plate, top with the chickpea mixture, spring onion (scallion) and drizzle over the dressing.

TIP

You could also try caramelising your onions in balsamic vinegar and agave for a sweeter, not-so-naughty taste! (Follow the method for caramelising pears on page 94.)

Avocado, Mango and Dill Salad

serves 1

30g (1¼oz) baby spinach leaves
1 tbsp olive oil
Pinch of sumac
Juice of 1 lime
¼ ripe avocado, diced
100g (3½oz) mango, diced
5g (¼oz) dill, chopped into
    1cm (½in) pieces
1 small garlic clove, grated
2.5cm (1in) piece of red chilli,
    finely sliced diagonally,
    to garnish
Sprouts, to garnish

You just can't beat a summer salad! This is delicious and doesn't leave you feeling at all bloated – ideal for those spring and summer months when you are wearing slightly lighter clothes!

Toss the baby spinach leaves with the olive oil, sumac and lime juice and arrange in a bowl.

Place the avocado and mango, most of the dill and the garlic in a separate bowl and mix together. Spoon onto the spinach and serve immediately, garnished with the chilli, sprouts and the remaining dill.

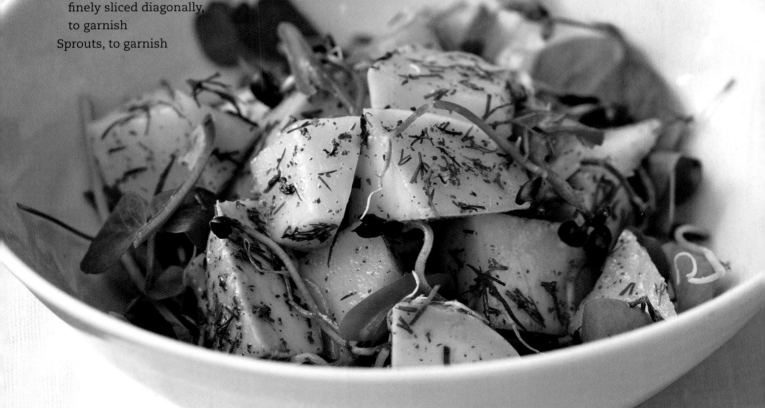

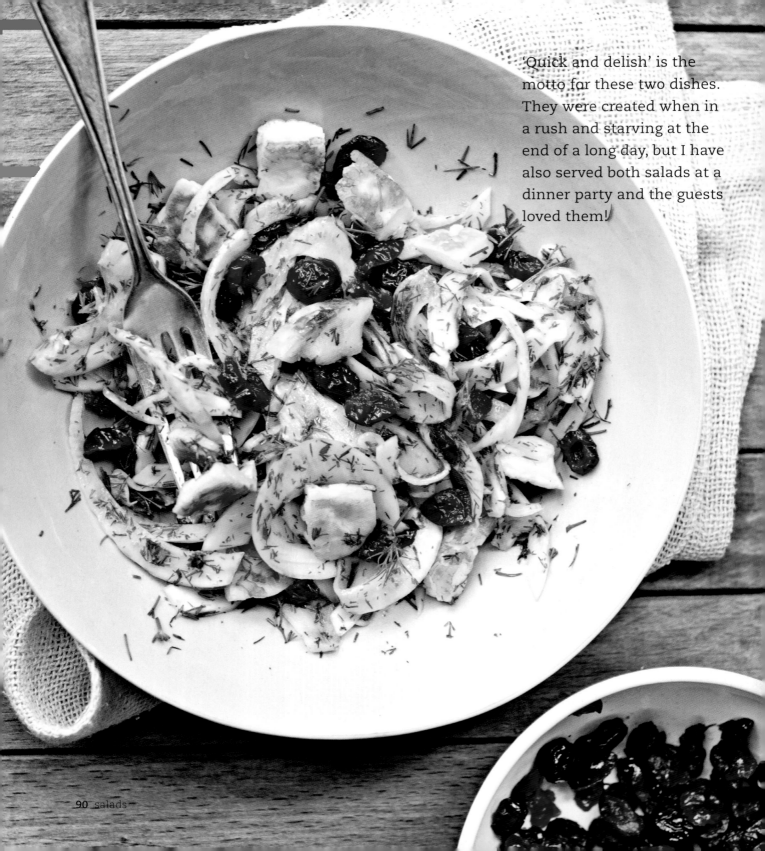

'Quick and delish' is the motto for these two dishes. They were created when in a rush and starving at the end of a long day, but I have also served both salads at a dinner party and the guests loved them!

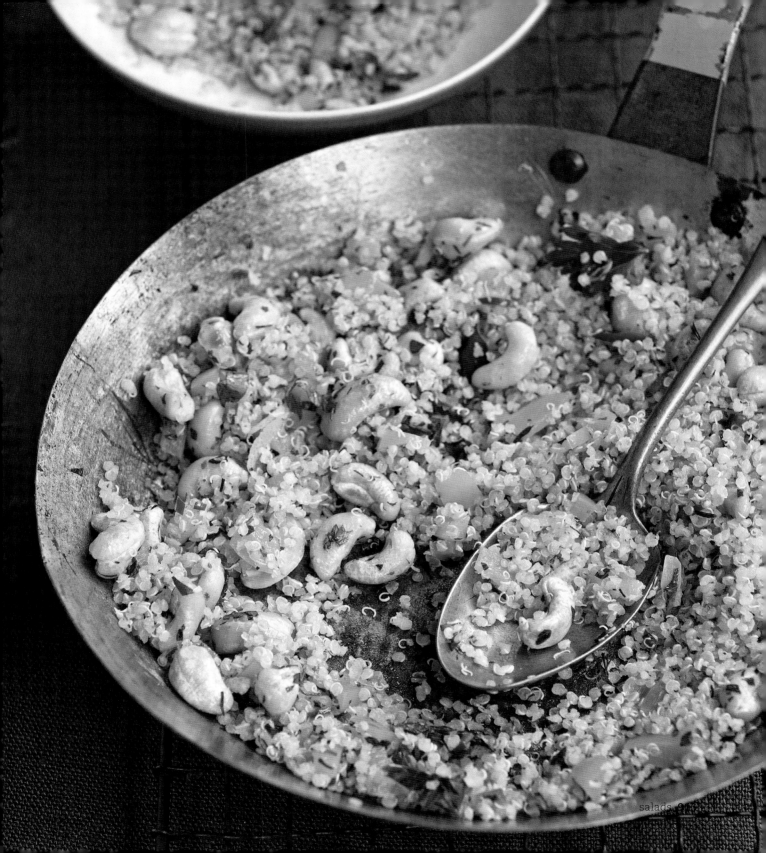

Fennel and Halloumi Salad

serves 2

150g (5oz) fennel, finely sliced

Juice of ½ lemon

2 tbsp olive oil

100g (3½oz) sheep's halloumi cheese, cut into small dice

1 small garlic clove, grated

50g (2oz/scant ½ cup) dried cranberries, soaked in warm water for 20 minutes and drained

15g (½oz) dill, chopped

(Pictured on page 90.) Halloumi – or 'squeaky cheese' (because it squeaks when you chew it) – is easy to cook, but a good tip is not to take your eye off it as it browns quickly and you want it golden, not burnt to a crisp.

Finely slice the fennel into a serving bowl and immediately toss it in the lemon juice to prevent oxidation.

Place a frying pan over a high heat, drizzle in the olive oil and reduce the heat to medium. Add the diced halloumi and cook for about 2 minutes on each side, until golden.

Add the garlic to the fennel and mix well. Stir in the cranberries and dill. Mix well and top with the warm halloumi.

Jewelled Quinoa

serves 1

40g (1½oz/scant ¼ cup) quinoa

1 tsp bouillon powder

2 tbsp olive oil

20g (¾oz) red onion, diced

1 garlic clove, finely chopped

Pinch of dried tarragon

½ yellow pepper, diced

¼ red chilli, finely diced

Zest and juice of ½ lemon

20g (¾oz/scant ¼ cup) raw cashews

15g (½oz) dried cranberries

20g (¾oz) flat-leaf parsley, finely chopped

25g (1oz) feta, crumbled

(Pictured on page 91.) Cook a batch of quinoa once a week, you can then warm it up in portions. Add pomegranate seeds for a burst of colour and freshness.

Measure the volume of the quinoa and bring twice the volume of water to the boil in a pan. Add the quinoa and bouillon powder, bring back to the boil, then simmer for 20 minutes, or until the 'germ' separates. Drain and set aside. Meanwhile soak the dried cranberries.

Heat the oil in a large pan, add the onion and garlic and sauté gently for 5 minutes, until softened, then add the tarragon and 2 tablespoons of water and cook for a further 2–3 minutes, until the onions are soft.

Stir in the yellow pepper, chilli, lemon juice, cashews and drained cranberries with another 2 tablespoons of water. Add the quinoa, stir to combine, and heat through for 2–3 minutes. Remove from the heat and stir in the grated lemon zest and chopped parsley. Stir in the crumbled feta and serve warm or cold, whichever you prefer.

Raw Nutty Coleslaw

serves 2 as a side dish

2 celery stalks
1 carrot, thinly sliced
    diagonally
50g (2oz/½ cup) mixed sprouts
    (such as mung beans, alfalfa,
    sunflower)

For the dressing
150g (5oz/1 cup) raw cashews
1 tsp English mustard
Juice of 1 lemon
About 125ml (4fl oz/½ cup)
    water

Instead of opting for the usual artery-clogging mayonnaise version, try coating your fresh, crunchy coleslaw vegetables in this delicious, creamy, high-protein healthy alternative.

Using a potato peeler, shred the celery into long spaghetti-like strips and place in a bowl with the carrot and sprouts.

Place the cashews, mustard and lemon juice in a blender with most of the water and blend to a smooth, creamy paste, adding more water a little at a time if necessary.

Add the dressing to the bowl and toss gently to combine.

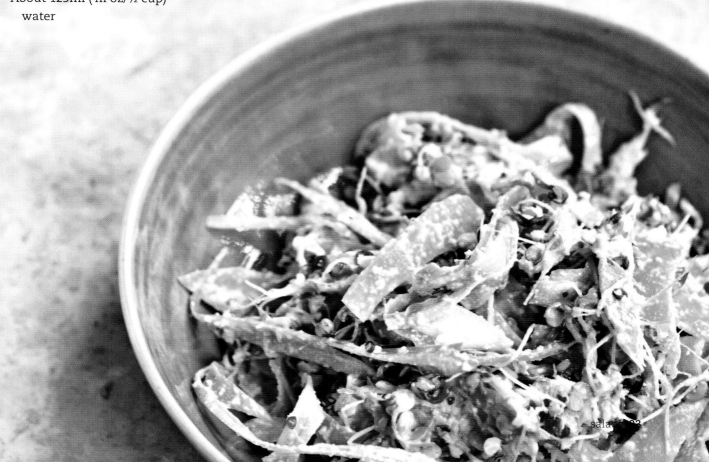

Caramelised Pear and Lentil Salad

serves 2

4 tbsp olive oil

1 tbsp agave syrup

1 tbsp balsamic vinegar

1 ripe pear, quartered and cored

30g (1¼oz/scant ¼ cup) Puy lentils

1 vine of baby tomatoes

20g (¾oz/scant ¼ cup) walnuts, soaked for 30 minutes, drained and broken into pieces

2 spring onions (scallions), thinly sliced diagonally

1 red chilli, thinly sliced diagonally

Juice of ½ lemon

60g (2½oz) rocket (arugula) leaves

I love this salad as it looks beautiful as well as tasting unbelievably good. I like my lentils al dente and slightly nutty tasting, but if you like them more mushy then extend the cooking time a little longer.

Place 2 tablespoons of the olive oil with the agave syrup and balsamic vinegar in a shallow pan, add the pear and half-cover the pan with a lid. Simmer for 30 minutes, or until the pear is caramelised all over. Check frequently to make sure there is enough liquid, adding water a tablespoon at a time if necessary.

Meanwhile, place the Puy lentils in a pan, cover with plenty of cold water, bring to the boil, then simmer for 20–25 minutes, until al dente; cook longer if you prefer them softer. Drain and set aside.

Preheat the oven to 160°C/325°F/gas mark 3. Place the tomatoes, still on their vine, on a baking tray (cookie sheet) and bake for 15 minutes, or until the skins soften and start to split.

Put the walnuts, spring onions (scallions) and chilli in a bowl, add the lentils, the remaining olive oil and the lemon juice, and toss gently.

To serve, arrange the rocket (arugula) leaves on 2 plates, pile the lentil salad on top and top with the pears and vine tomatoes.

NUTRITIONAL NUGGET
Puy lentils are a great source of zinc and magnesium, to support you in stressful times.

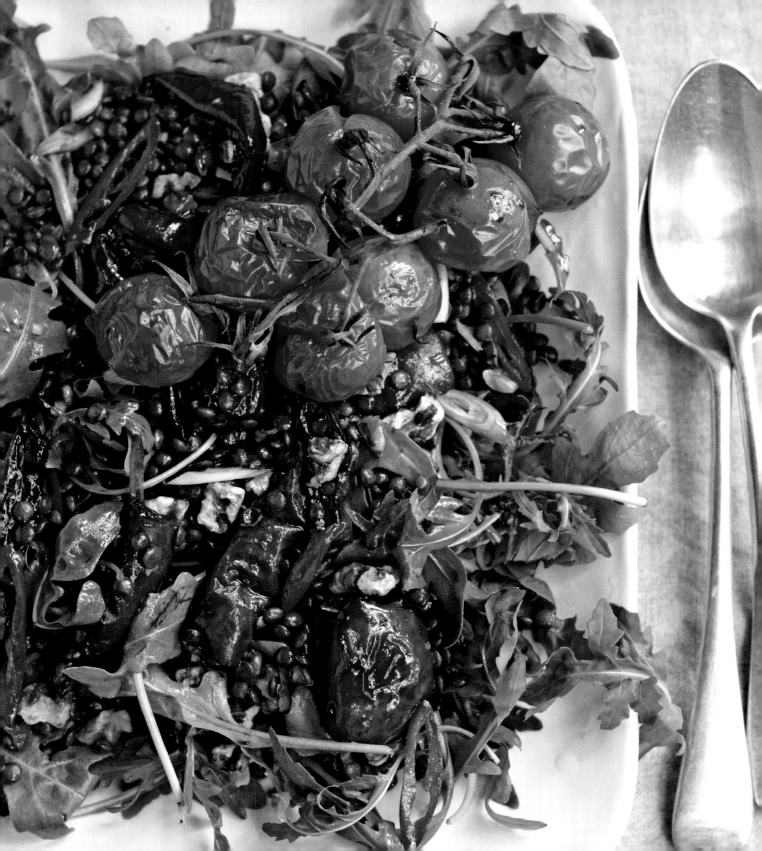

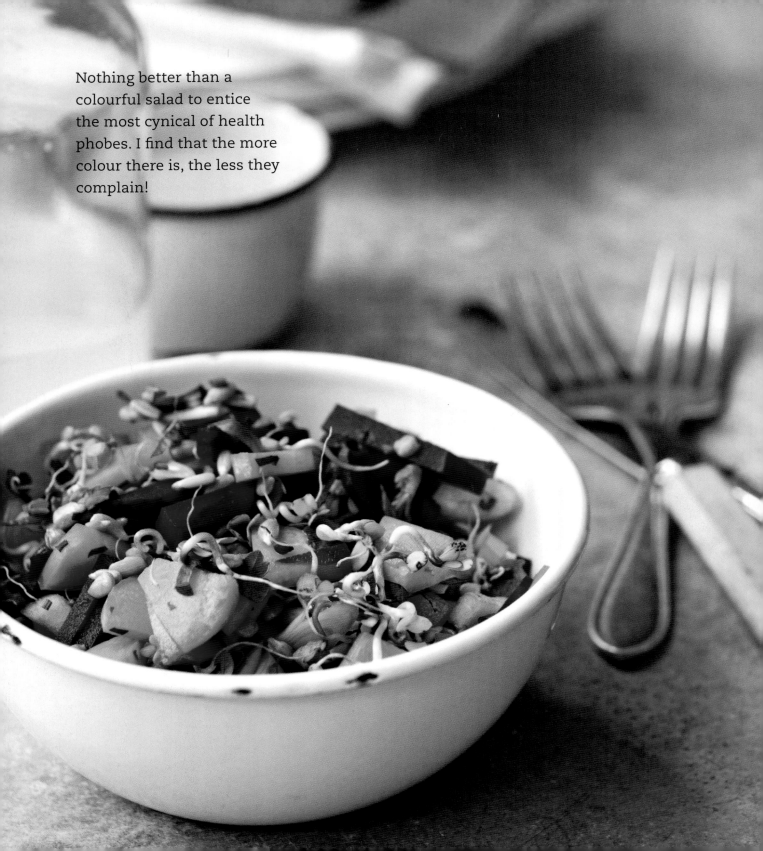

Nothing better than a colourful salad to entice the most cynical of health phobes. I find that the more colour there is, the less they complain!

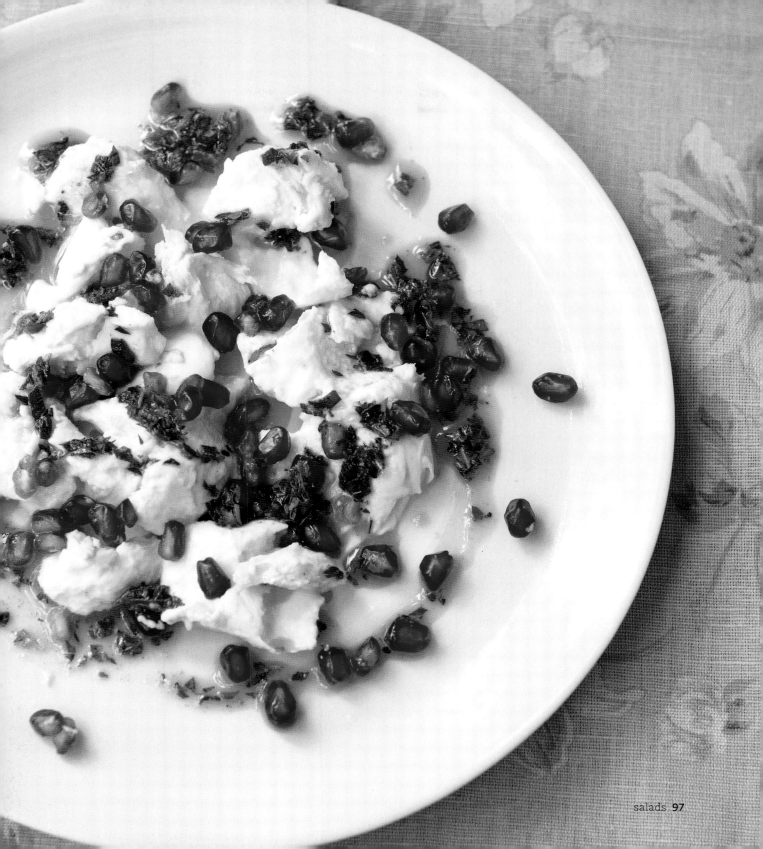

Roots and Walnut Salad

serves 1 as a main dish or
   serves 2 as a side dish

15g (½oz/scant ¼ cup) raw
   walnuts, chopped in quarters
50g (2oz) beetroot (beet)
75g (3oz) carrot
20g (¾oz) pear
1 spring onion (scallion)
1 tbsp extra virgin olive oil
1 tbsp tamari
Pinch of cayenne pepper
15g (½oz) coriander (cilantro)

(Pictured on page 96.) Beetroot (beet) is great for supporting the liver in its natural detoxification processes, and walnuts contain essential fats that feed the brain (it looks like two halves of the brain itself!).

An hour before you want to assemble your salad soak the walnuts. Next, peel the beetroot (beet), finely slice it and pop into a bowl. Dice the carrot and pear and finely slice the spring onion (scallion). Tip into the bowl along with the soaked walnuts. Drizzle in the olive oil and tamari, sprinkle in the cayenne pepper and mix gently.

Chop the coriander (cilantro) leaves and stir in just before serving with a garnish of beautiful sprouts.

Pomegranate and Mozzarella Salad

serves 2

Seeds from 1 ruby red
   pomegranate
2 balls of mozzarella

For the dressing
2 tbsp roughly chopped flat-
   leaf parsley and mint
1 garlic clove, grated
1 red chilli, deseeded and
   finely chopped
2 tbsp extra virgin olive oil
Pinch of ground cumin

(Pictured on page 97.) I find the easiest way to get pomegranate seeds out of their pods is to loosen the seeds from their pith, then allow them to drop into a big bowl of cold water; the pith floats to the surface.

Remove the seeds from the pomegranate, following my method above or using your own technique.

Drain the mozzarella balls and tear into smallish pieces (about 6–8) and arrange on 2 plates, then blend the dressing ingredients with a hand-held blender or whisk together with a fork.

To serve, drizzle the dressing over the mozzarella, then sprinkle with the pomegranate seeds.

Pulsed Broad Bean and Pearl Barley Salad

serves 1

40g (1½oz/scant ¼ cup) pearl barley
1 tsp bouillon powder
30g (1¼oz) broad (fava) beans
2 tbsp olive oil
Juice of ½ lime

Pinch of Himalayan pink salt
1 small garlic clove
1 carrot, grated
15g (½oz) dill, finely chopped
Pinch of ground cumin
2 tenderstem broccoli stalks
½ red chilli, finely sliced diagonally, to garnish (optional)

The combination of beans and grain here provides all eight essential amino acids for building and repairing the whole body.

Place the pearl barley and bouillon powder in a pan, add plenty of cold water, bring to the boil, then simmer for 25–30 minutes, until tender. Drain and set aside.

Place the broad (fava) beans in a blender with the olive oil, lime juice and a pinch of salt, grate in the garlic and pulse for 1 minute to form a rough paste.

Transfer the pulsed beans to a bowl and stir in the pearl barley with the carrot, dill and a pinch of cumin.

Meanwhile, steam the broccoli until just tender.

Serve the pulsed bean mixture with the broccoli on top, garnished with sliced red chilli if you like.

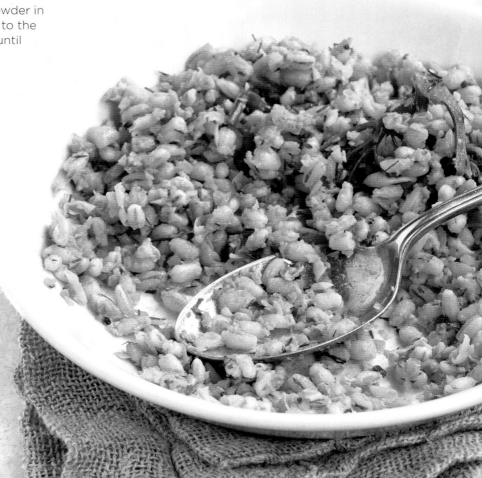

Portobello Mushroom and Fennel Salad

serves 1

1 portobello mushroom
1 garlic clove, finely sliced
3 sprigs of thyme
Pinch of Himalayan pink salt
2 tbsp olive oil
85g (3¼oz) fennel
Juice of ½ lemon
½ tbsp raw pumpkin seeds
5g (¼oz) flat-leaf parsley,
   roughly chopped

The combination of soft-textured mushroom and crisp, cool fennel with the slight bitterness of the pumpkin seeds reaches almost every part of the palate.

Preheat the oven to 180°C/350°F/gas mark 4.

Place the mushroom on a baking tray (cookie sheet) and sprinkle with the garlic, thyme and a pinch of salt, then drizzle over 1 tablespoon of the olive oil. Bake for 15 minutes, until tender.

Meanwhile, finely dice the fennel and toss with the remaining olive oil and the lemon juice.

To serve, place the mushroom on a plate, top with the fennel and sprinkle with the pumpkin seeds and chopped parsley.

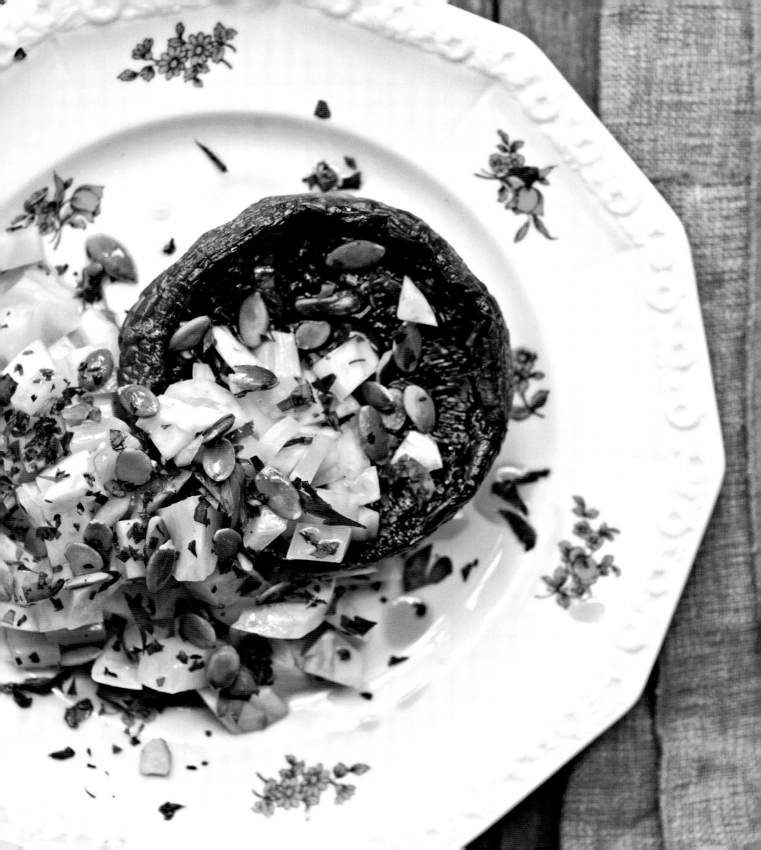

Beetroot, Roasted Garlic and Quinoa Salad with Feta

serves 2

♥ ♥ ♥

1 whole garlic bulb

1 large beetroot (beet), washed and cut into eighths or 2 small beetroot (beet), quartered

1 red onion, unpeeled and cut into eighths

4 tbsp olive oil

1 long vine of baby tomatoes

70g (2¾oz/generous ⅓ cup) quinoa

1 tsp bouillon powder

Pinch of Himalayan pink salt

40g (1½oz) mixed salad leaves (salad greens)

40g (1½oz) feta

Lemony Dressing or My Secret Salad Dressing (see page 104), to serve

NUTRITIONAL NUGGET

The beta-carotene found in beetroot, red tomatoes and red onion are all highly protective for your outer and inner skin. This is a great antioxidant salad for any time of the year.

The combination of textures and flavours in this dish makes my mouth water just thinking about it – contrast is the key ingredient here.

Preheat the oven to 170°C/340°F/gas mark 3½.

Chop the top off the garlic bulb so the cloves are slightly exposed and place on a baking tray (cookie sheet) with the beetroot (beet) and onion. Drizzle over 2 tablespoons of the olive oil and roast for 35 minutes. Add the tomatoes, still on their vine, and cook for a further 5–7 minutes, until softened.

Meanwhile, measure the volume of the quinoa and bring twice the volume of water to the boil in a pan. Add the quinoa and bouillon powder, bring back to the boil, then simmer for 20 minutes, or until the 'germ' separates. Drain and set aside.

When the vegetables are cooked, hold the base of the garlic bulb in a cloth, squeeze out the soft flesh onto a chopping board and mash it with a flat knife. Using the back of a tablespoon, very gently spread the mashed garlic over the quinoa to avoid clumping, then mix it in thoroughly. Stir in the remaining olive oil and a pinch of salt.

To serve, arrange the salad leaves (salad greens) on 2 plates and top with the quinoa. Scatter the beetroot (beet) and red onion around the edge, crumble over the feta and top with the vine tomatoes and your choice of dressing.

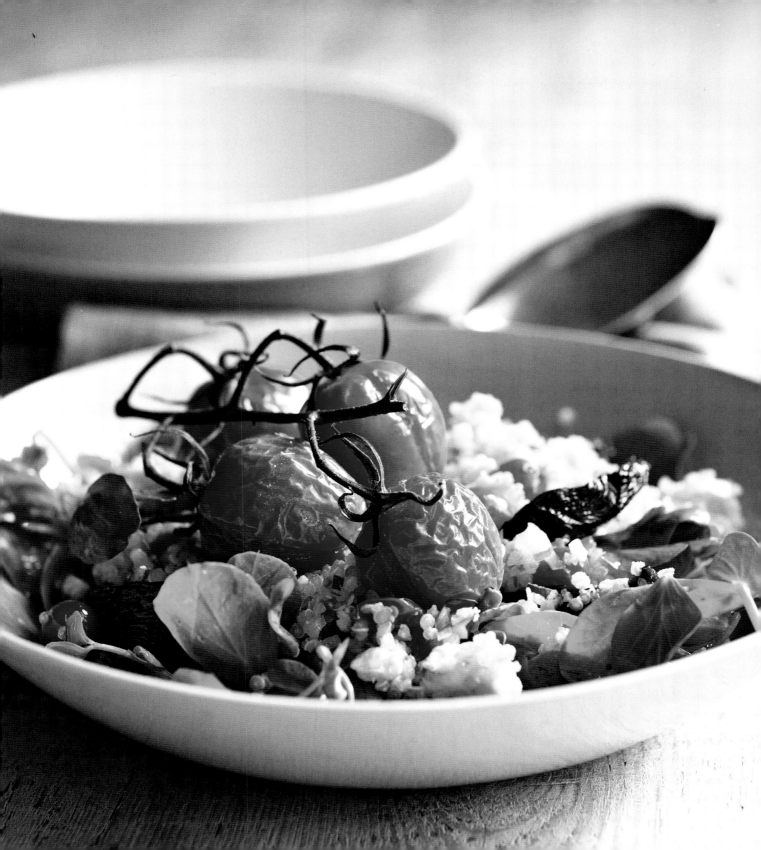

Five Salad Dressings

My Secret Salad Dressing

4 tbsp olive oil
2 tbsp tamari
2 tbsp balsamic vinegar
1 tbsp agave syrup

Simply mix together and drizzle over an eagerly awaiting salad!

Lemony Dressing

4 tbsp olive oil
2 tbsp apple cider vinegar
Juice of 1 lemon
1 small handful of coriander (cilantro)
1 tbsp agave syrup

Blend with a hand-held blender or in a mini food processor until creamy.

Tangy Almond Dressing

1 heaped tbsp almond butter
3 tbsp olive oil
Finely grated zest and juice of 1 lime
1 tbsp tamari
Pinch of cayenne pepper
1cm (½in) red chilli, deseeded and finely chopped

Blend with a hand-held blender or in a mini food processor until smooth.

Soya Mayonnaise Dressing

1 heaped tbsp soya yogurt
1 tbsp olive oil
1 small garlic clove, grated

Stir all the ingredients together until thoroughly combined.

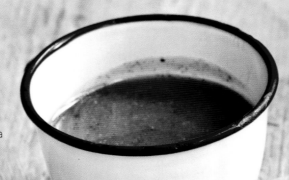

Clockwise from left
Choose from Tangy Almond, Lemony, My Secret Salad, Tahini and Cumin, or Soya Mayonnaise salad dressings.

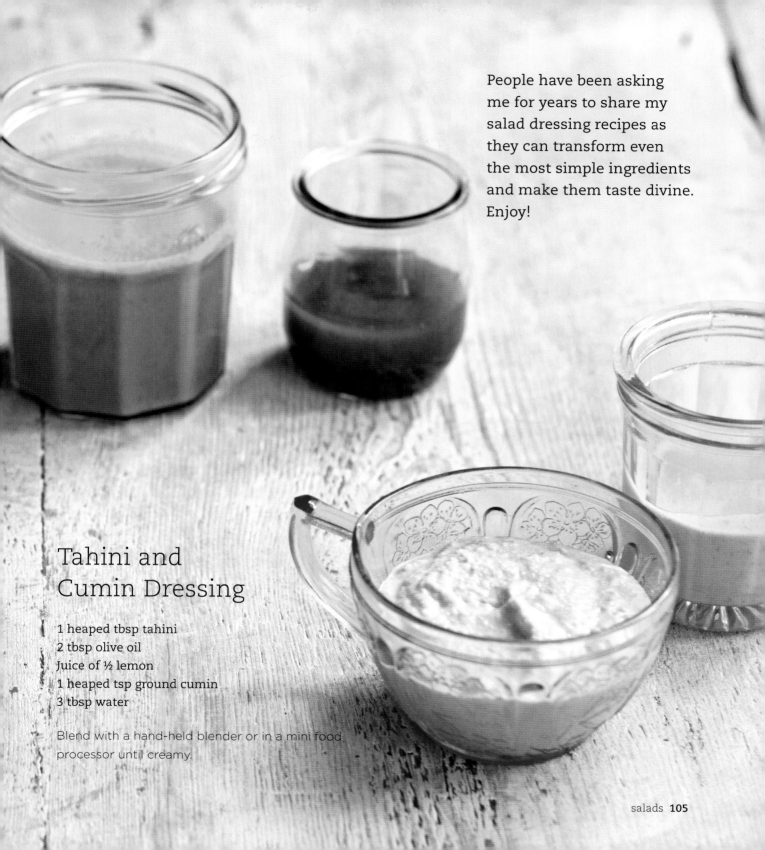

People have been asking me for years to share my salad dressing recipes as they can transform even the most simple ingredients and make them taste divine. Enjoy!

Tahini and Cumin Dressing

1 heaped tbsp tahini
2 tbsp olive oil
Juice of ½ lemon
1 heaped tsp ground cumin
3 tbsp water

Blend with a hand-held blender or in a mini food processor until creamy.

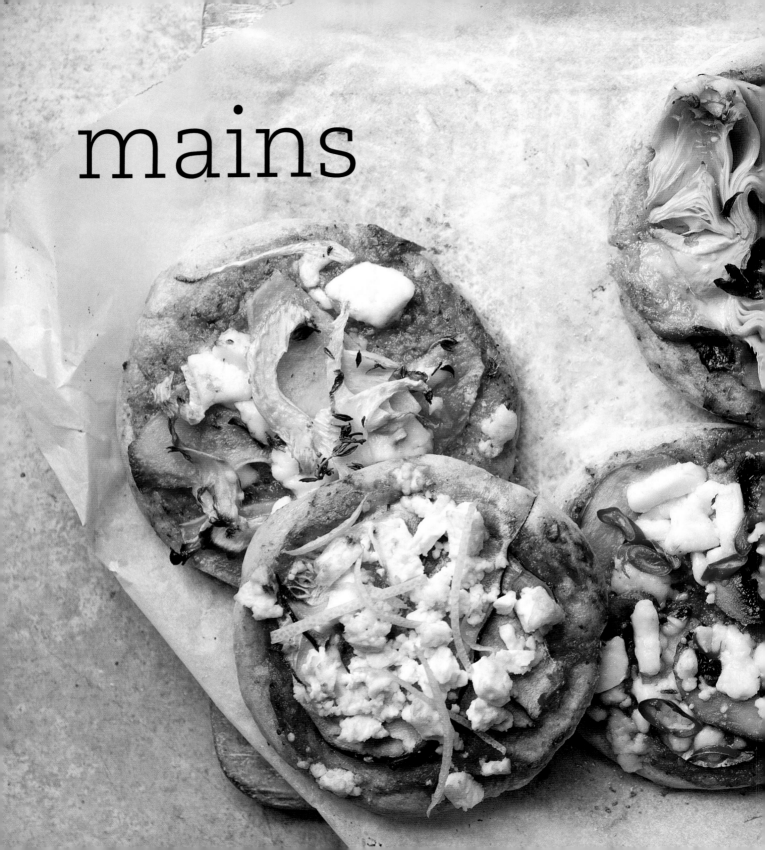

mains

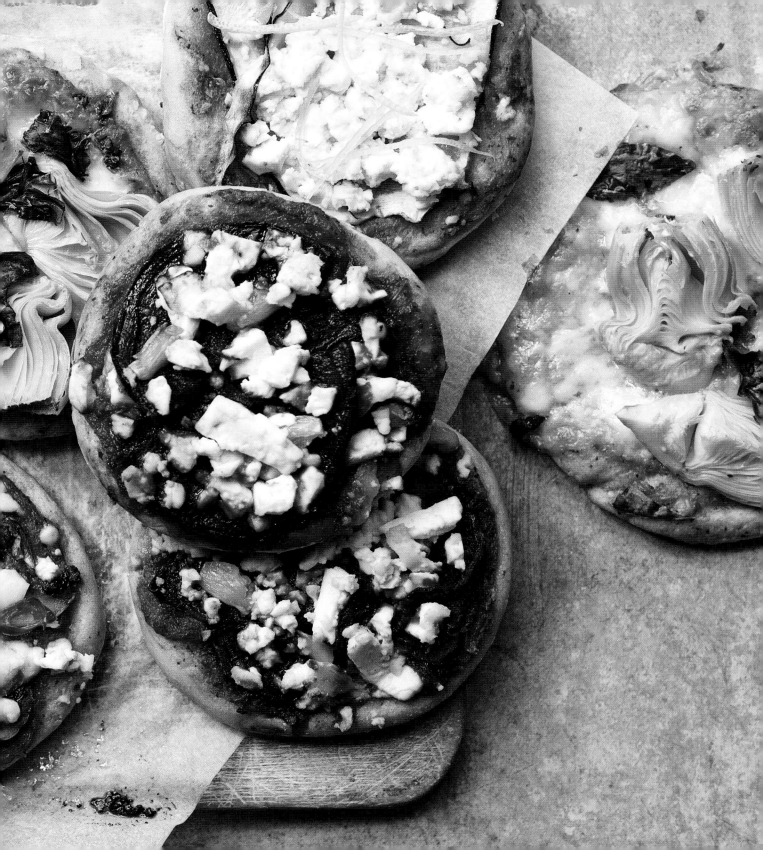

Mini Pizzas

makes 8

For the bases
½ tsp active dry yeast
170ml (6fl oz/⅔ cup) lukewarm
    water
285g (9¼oz/2¼ cups) white
    spelt flour
½ tsp Himalayan pink salt

For the sauce
1 tbsp olive oil
1 onion, chopped
1 garlic clove
2 tbsp capers, rinsed and
    drained
Pinch of dried chilli flakes
300g (10oz) tomatoes, deseeded
    and diced
1 tbsp fresh or
    1 tsp dried oregano

(Pictured on pages 106–107.) My mother could never eat pizza because of a wheat intolerance, so it's been my mission to put pizza on her plate. And here it is! (The pizza toppings recipes opposite are per mini pizza, so double or quadruple up, as necessary.)

Preheat the oven to 200°C/400°F/gas mark 6. Mix the yeast with the water, cover and set aside in a warm room for about 15 minutes.

Meanwhile, make the pizza sauce by heating the oil in a pan and sautéing the onion and garlic gently until the onions start to go soft, then add a splash of water to cool and add the remaining ingredients. Simmer for 15 minutes until the right consistency.

Whisk the yeast and water mixture and leave for another 5 minutes.

Place the flour and salt in a large bowl. Make a well in the centre and pour in the yeast mixture. Turn out onto a work surface and knead for 5-10 minutes until smooth and silky to the touch, adding a little more flour if necessary.

Divide the bread dough into pieces, roll each piece into a ball, place on a baking tray (cookie sheet) lined with baking parchment and flatten into a circle. Smear on some tomato sauce followed by your choice of toppings (see opposite), then bake for 5 minutes, rotate and bake for a further 5 minutes, or until ready.

NUTRITIONAL NUGGET
Spelt is an ancient wheat-based grain that is far lower in gluten than most modern wheats. The mineral content is far richer and much less processed. Many people who have a wheat intolerance are able to tolerate spelt.

Artichoke and Basil with Mozzarella

2 canned artichoke hearts, thinly
  sliced
2 basil leaves, shredded
20g (¾oz) buffalo mozzarella, torn
  into small pieces

Courgette and Lemon with Feta

15g (½oz) courgette (zucchini), thinly sliced
3 strips of lemon rind, finely sliced
15g (½oz) feta, crumbled

Fennel and Sweet Potato with Goat's Cheese

10g (½oz) fennel, thinly sliced
15g (½oz) sweet potato, thinly sliced
6g (¼oz) hard goat's cheese, grated

Roasted Garlic, Beetroot and Feta

3 garlic cloves, roasted and squeezed
  out of the skins
7g (¼oz) beetroot (beet), thinly sliced
10g (½oz) feta, crumbled

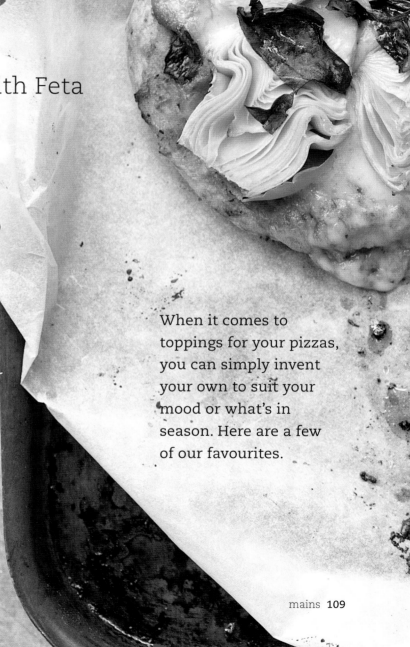

When it comes to toppings for your pizzas, you can simply invent your own to suit your mood or what's in season. Here are a few of our favourites.

Spanish Omelette with Dill and Sweet Potato

serves 4

200g (7oz) sweet potato, quartered lengthways and thinly sliced

2 tbsp olive oil, plus extra for greasing

6 eggs

30g (1¼oz) red pepper, deseeded and cut into strips

2 tbsp finely chopped dill

Pinch of Himalayan pink salt

Mixed leaf salad, to serve

For variations, add

60g (2½oz) sliced leeks

100g (3½oz) asparagus

NUTRITIONAL NUGGET
For vegetarians, eggs are one of the only sources of complete protein and fortunately do not, as previously thought, cause cholesterol levels to rise.

This is what I always make when I'm 'too tired to cook' as it's so simple to prepare and gives me so much energy. Add some thinly sliced leeks or a few asparagus spears for even more flavour and texture.

Preheat the oven to 170°C/340°F/gas mark 3½.

Arrange the sweet potato slices on a baking tray (cookie sheet), drizzle with the olive oil and bake for 20 minutes, until tender. Leave the oven switched on.

Beat the eggs in a large bowl and add the sweet potato slices, red pepper, dill and a pinch of salt.

Using a sheet of kitchen paper (paper towel), coat a non-stick ovenproof frying pan evenly with olive oil. Heat over a low heat, then pour in the egg mixture and cook, loosening the edge of the omelette with a spatula every 30 seconds to make sure it doesn't stick. When the eggs have set to about 5mm (¼in) from the edge of the pan, transfer the frying pan to the oven and cook for 15–20 minutes. To test whether the omelette is cooked, press the top with a palette knife – no egg should ooze out.

Serve warm or cold with a mixed leaf salad.

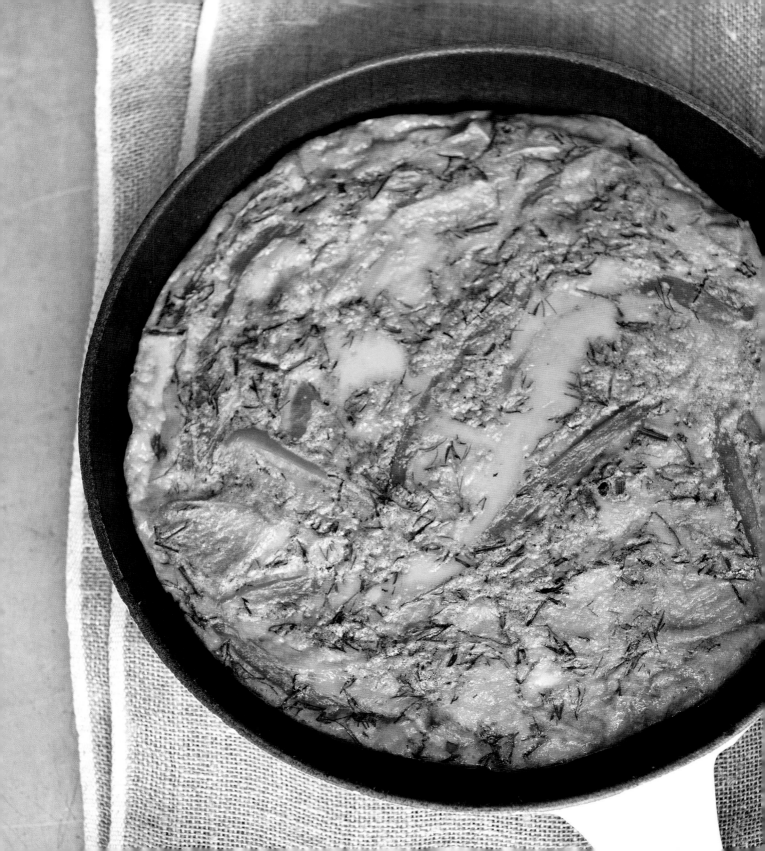

Layered Vegetable Bake

serves 4

80g (3oz/scant ½ cup) Puy
   lentils
4 tbsp olive oil, plus extra for
   brushing
1 beef tomato, roughly chopped
1 garlic clove, sliced
1 beetroot (beet), cut into
   small dice
½ tsp tamari
1 tsp dried, chopped chives
Pinch of ground cumin
2 tbsp water
400g (13oz) butternut squash,
   thinly sliced lengthways
300g (10oz) courgettes
   (zucchini), thinly sliced
   lengthways

This knocks the socks off any traditional lasagne I've ever tasted! Instead of the usual pasta layers I have used colourful vegetables, so it leaves you feeling much, much lighter but totally satisfied.

Preheat the oven to 170°C/340°F/gas mark 3½.

Place the lentils in a small pan, cover with water, bring to the boil, then simmer for 10–15 minutes, until al dente. Drain and set aside.

Meanwhile, heat the olive oil in a large pan and squash the tomato into the oil to make a base for the sauce. Add the garlic and beetroot (beet) with the tamari, chives and a pinch of cumin. Add the water and cook over a medium heat for 15 minutes, or until reduced to a thick sauce. Add the lentils to the pan with a splash more water and simmer for a further 5 minutes.

Layer half the butternut squash and a third of the courgettes (zucchini) in an ovenproof dish and spread over half the lentil sauce. Repeat the layers, finishing with the remaining courgettes (zucchini). Brush the courgettes (zucchini) generously with olive oil, then bake for 45 minutes, or until the vegetables are just tender.

You may also like to try using the parsley oil from the Pomegranate and Mozzarella Salad (see page 98) instead of olive oil on the top.

WHAT IS TAMARI?
This is a wheat-free soy sauce substitute. Like soy sauce, it has a rich flavour and is dark; it's excellent in dressings and marinades.

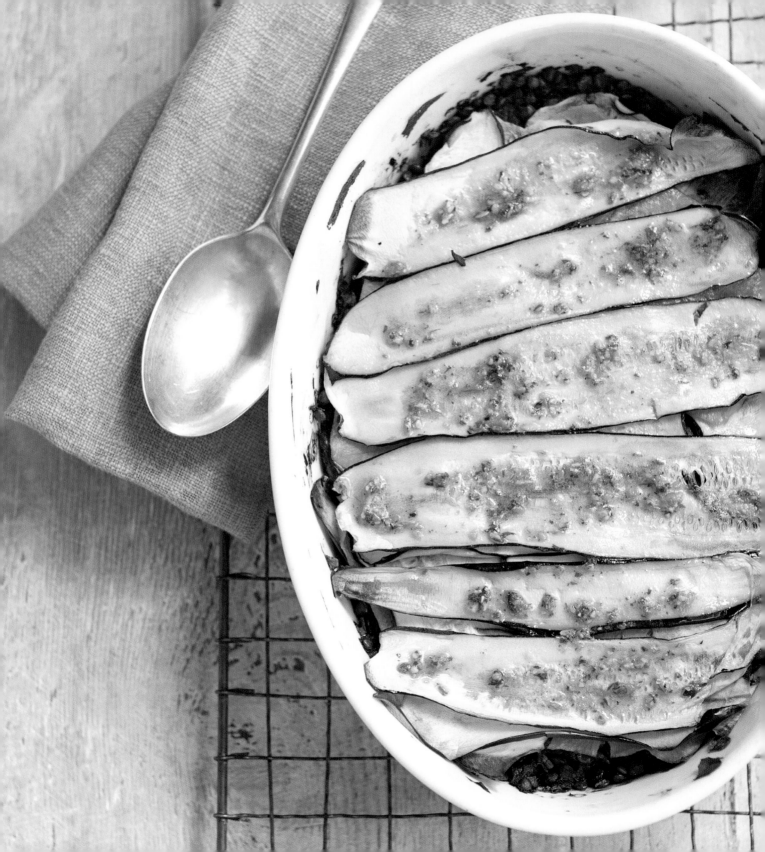

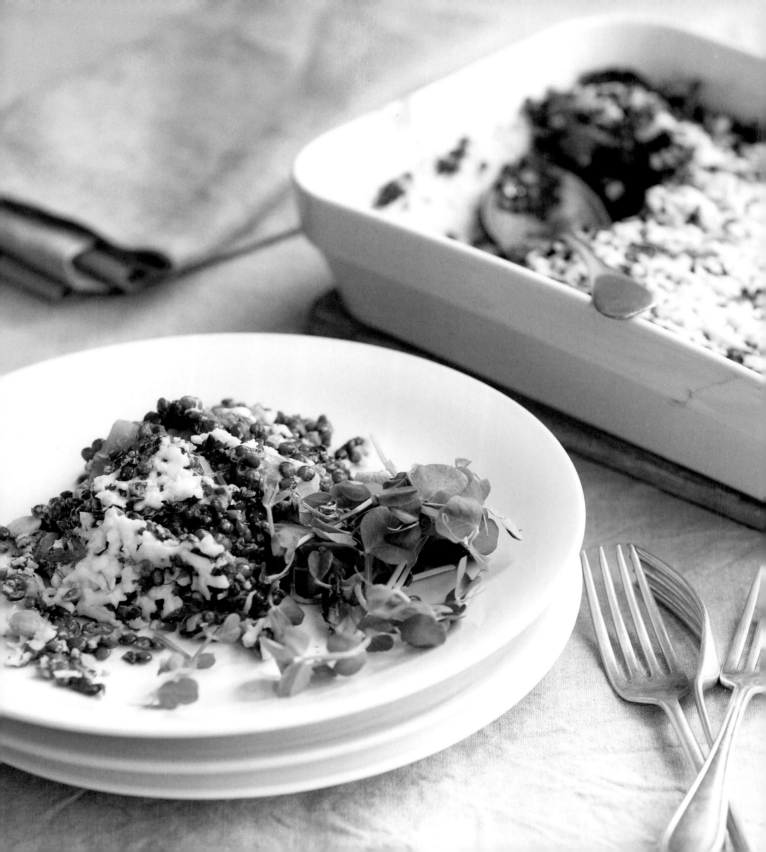

Puy Lentil, Coconut and Goat's Cheese Bake

serves 4

125g (4oz/scant ⅔ cup) Puy lentils

100g (3½oz) butternut squash, diced

3 tbsp olive oil

2 garlic cloves

200ml (7fl oz/generous ¾ cup) coconut milk

80g (3oz) goat's Cheddar, grated

40g (1½oz) flat-leaf parsley, chopped, to garnish

½ red chilli, finely sliced, to garnish

Watercress, to serve

For those who are craving a richer dish, bake away! To make lentils easier to digest, when boiling them from scratch pop a piece of kombu seaweed into the pan as this will help break down the fibre in the lentils.

Preheat the oven to 170°C/340°F/gas mark 3½.

Place the lentils in a small pan, cover with water, bring to the boil, then simmer for 10–15 minutes, until al dente. Drain and set aside.

Place the diced butternut squash on a baking tray (cookie sheet), drizzle with 2 tablespoons of the olive oil and bake for 10 minutes, until nearly tender. Leave the oven switched on.

Meanwhile, heat the remaining olive oil in a pan and sauté the garlic until softened. Stir in the lentils and squash with 50ml (2fl oz/scant ¼ cup) of the coconut milk and leave to simmer for 5 minutes.

Pour the mixture into an ovenproof baking dish or 4 individual ramekins, pour over the remaining coconut milk and bake for 15 minutes. Sprinkle over the grated goat's Cheddar and return to the oven to melt the cheese.

Serve with some watercress and sprinkled with chopped parsley and the sliced chilli if you like a bit of heat.

Quinoa and Cranberry Burgers

serves 4

100g (3½oz) sweet potato, chopped

3 tbsp olive oil

100g (3½oz/½ cup) quinoa

2 tsp bouillon powder

40g (1½oz/⅓ cup) dried cranberries, soaked in water for 4 hours and drained

7g (¼oz) parsley, chopped

2 heaped tbsp nutritional yeast flakes

15g (½oz) arrowroot flour

Pinch of Himalayan pink salt

1 egg white

Olive oil, for sautéing

For the sauce

50g (2oz/⅓ cup) macadamia nuts

2 tsp tahini

1 tsp grated fresh root ginger

Juice of 1 lemon

2 tbsp water

Pinch of cayenne pepper

Pinch of ground cumin

These sweet yet savoury mini burgers could be your main dish, or even make them bite-size for canapés. If you don't have nutritional yeast flakes, don't worry, but they do add extra vitamin B12 and a slight cheesy taste.

To make the sauce, place all the sauce ingredients in a blender, whizz until smooth and set aside.

Preheat the oven to 170°C/340°F/gas mark 3½.

Place the chopped sweet potato on a baking tray (cookie sheet), drizzle with 2 tablespoons of the olive oil and bake for 30 minutes, until tender. Transfer to a mini food processor (or use a hand-held blender) with the remaining olive oil and blend to a purée. Increase the oven temperature to 180°C/350°F/gas mark 4.

Meanwhile, measure the volume of the quinoa and bring twice the volume of water to the boil in a pan. Add the quinoa and bouillon powder, bring back to the boil, then simmer for 20 minutes, or until the 'germ' separates. Drain and set aside.

Place the sweet potato purée in a bowl with the quinoa and the remaining ingredients and mix to a sticky consistency. Form the mixture into 8 burgers.

Heat a little olive oil in a frying pan and, working in batches if necessary, cook the burgers for about 2 minutes on each side, until golden. Transfer to a baking tray (cookie sheet) lined with baking parchment and bake for 10 minutes.

Serve the burgers at once, with the sauce.

WHAT IS HIMALAYAN PINK SALT?
This delicately pink crystalline salt originates from ancient seas. It's naturally dried by the sun and is totally pure and full of amazing minerals.

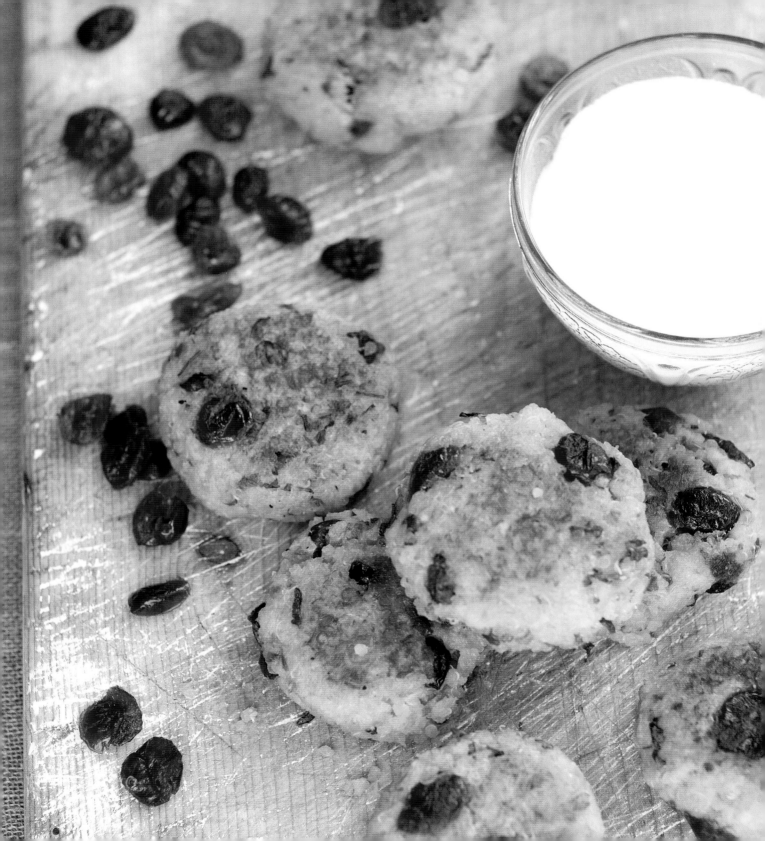

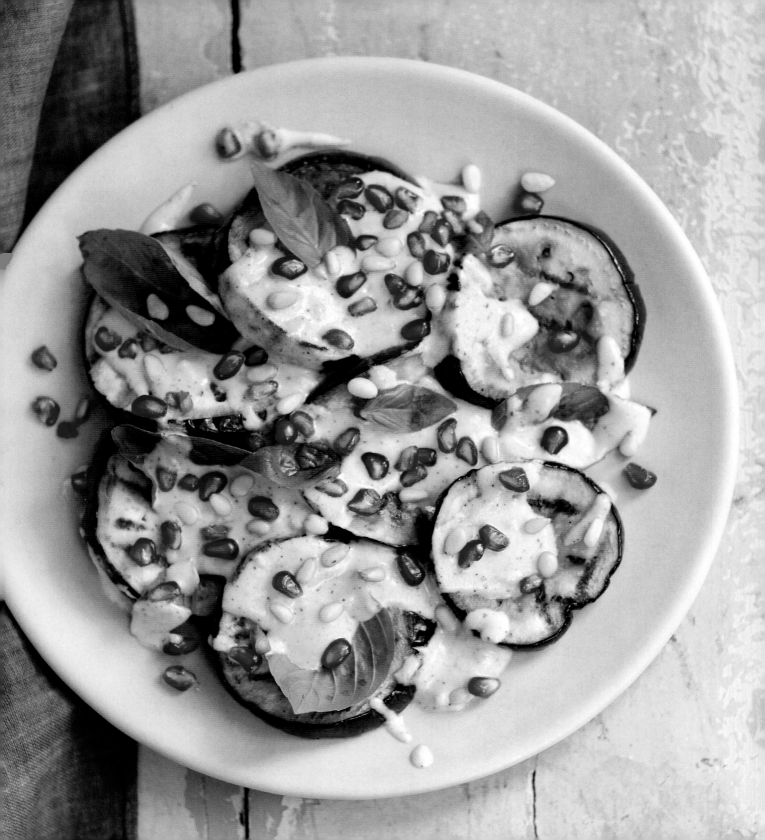

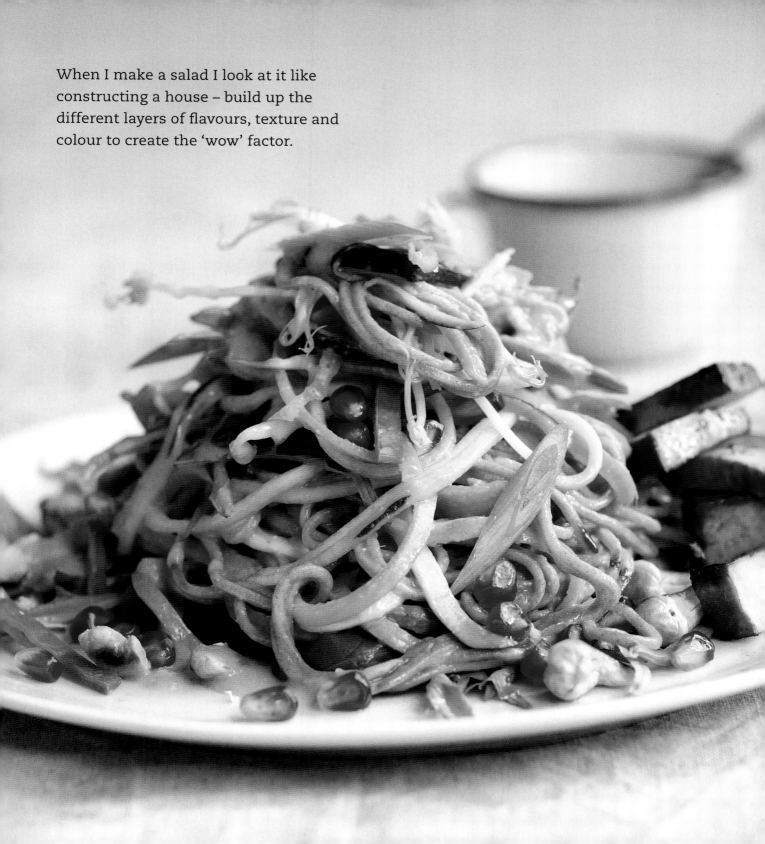

When I make a salad I look at it like constructing a house – build up the different layers of flavours, texture and colour to create the 'wow' factor.

Roasted Aubergine with Sumac and Tahini Dressing

serves 4

2 aubergines (eggplant), cut
widthways into 1cm (½in)
slices
Olive oil, for brushing
2 tbsp pine nuts, toasted
Large handful of basil leaves
Seeds from ½ pomegranate
(see page 98 for how to
remove them from the pod)
Himalayan pink salt
Freshly ground black pepper

For the dressing
40g (1½oz/generous ⅛ cup)
tahini
3 tbsp extra virgin
olive oil
3 tbsp lemon juice
4 tbsp hot water
1 garlic clove, crushed
1 tsp sumac
Himalayan pink salt

(Pictured on page 118.) This Lebanese-influenced dish tastes lighter than most aubergine (eggplant) dishes from that region. The sumac has a sharp lemon flavour and is a key ingredient in Middle Eastern cooking.

To make the dressing, place all the ingredients in a bowl and whisk until smooth. Taste and adjust the seasoning if necessary, then chill until required (the sauce can be stored in the fridge for up to 3 days).

Lightly brush both sides of the aubergine (eggplant) slices with olive oil and sprinkle with salt and black pepper.

Grill on both sides on a very hot griddle pan until soft and golden. Alternatively, roast for 20–30 minutes in a preheated oven, 220°C/425°F/gas mark 7. (This can also be done up to 3 days in advance – store the roasted aubergine (eggplant) slices in the fridge, but bring to room temperature before serving.)

To serve, arrange the roasted aubergine (eggplant) slices on a serving dish, slightly overlapping. Drizzle with the dressing and sprinkle with toasted pine nuts, basil leaves and pomegranate seeds.

TIP
When you add the water to the tahini and start to stir it will look like its curdling but fret not – just keep whisking and it will become smooth.

Noodle and Smoked Tofu Salad with Mirin Dressing

serves 2

For the salad

125g (4oz) buckwheat noodles

50g (2oz) carrot

30g (1¼oz) courgette (zucchini)

20g (¾oz) daikon, thinly sliced

20g (¾oz) mangetout (snow peas), thinly sliced

20g (¾oz) mizuna leaves

20g (¾oz/¼ cup) beansprouts

50g (2oz) pomegranate seeds, plus extra to garnish

4 tsp sesame oil

125g (4oz) smoked tofu, cut into 6 chunky squares

2 tsp tamari

Coriander (cilantro) leaves

Sushi ginger

50g (2oz/⅓ cup) dry roasted cashews, to garnish

For the dressing

25g (1oz) white miso paste

25ml (1fl oz/2 tbsp) mirin

2 tsp sesame oil

2 tsp umeboshi plum purée

125g (4oz) sushi ginger

½ tbsp rice wine vinegar

1 tbsp lime juice

75ml (3fl oz/scant ⅓ cup) olive oil

2 tsp water

(Pictured on page 119.) This distinctly Asian recipe is both delicious and beautiful to behold, with the carrot and courgette (zucchini) spirals. The buckwheat (soba) noodles add a hearty feel to the dish.

To make the dressing, whizz all the ingredients in a blender until thick and smooth.

Use a spiraliser to make carrot and courgette (zucchini) spirals. Cook the noodles according to the packet instructions, then rinse in cold water and drain well. Place in a bowl with the carrot and courgette (zucchini) spirals and mix well. Mix in the remaining vegetables, pomegranate seeds and 2 teaspoons of the sesame oil.

Just before serving, heat the remaining sesame oil in a frying pan. Add the tofu and cook for 2 minutes, until brown on all sides. Add the tamari, toss to coat and glaze the tofu, and cook for 2 minutes. Thread onto 2 wooden skewers, layering the tofu cubes with whole coriander (cilantro) leaves and sushi ginger.

To serve, add the dressing to the noodles and toss gently to coat. Arrange a heap of salad on each plate and scatter with roasted cashews and pomegranate seeds, then sit a tofu skewer at one side.

NUTRITIONAL NUGGET
In spite of its name, buckwheat is not related to wheat and, like quinoa, is classed as a pseudocereal. Buckwheat is particularly high in rutin, which strengthens and protects the delicate lining of our capillaries and arteries – this is a heart-healthy meal.

Sweetcorn and Broad Bean Fritters

serves 2

2 large eggs

100g (3½oz/scant ⅔ cup) frozen sweetcorn, defrosted and drained

115g (3¾oz) frozen baby broad (fava) beans, defrosted and drained

50g (2oz/⅓ cup) rice flour

2 tbsp finely chopped coriander (cilantro)

1 bird's eye chilli (Thai chilli), deseeded and finely chopped

Juice of 1 lime

¼ tsp Himalayan pink salt

Freshly ground black pepper

Sunflower oil, for sautéing

For the dressing

2 tsp white miso

1 tsp agave syrup

1 tsp lemon juice

These colourful fritters are unbelievably delicious. They give you the impression of being substantial and really rather naughty, but leave you feeling light and bright.

To make the dressing, whisk the ingredients together and set aside.

To make the fritters, whisk the eggs in a large bowl and add the sweetcorn and broad (fava) beans. Add the flour and stir well to combine. Add the coriander (cilantro) and chilli with the lime juice, season with the salt and plenty of black pepper, and stir in.

Heat a little sunflower oil in a large frying pan and, working in batches, cook spoonfuls of the mixture on both sides, until golden. Depending on the size you want, use 1 or 2 tablespoons of mixture for each fritter.

Serve the fritters with the Feta, Cucumber and Spinach Salad (see opposite) and accompanied with the dressing.

NUTRITIONAL NUGGET
Sweetcorn is one of the highest sources of vitamin D – so not only do they look sunny, they are!

Feta, Cucumber and Spinach Salad

serves 4

½ tsp bouillon powder

6 tenderstem broccoli stalks

40g (1½oz/⅓ cup) frozen peas, defrosted

1 small yellow pepper, deseeded and diced

1 spring onion (scallion), finely sliced diagonally

60g (2½oz) cucumber, diced

5cm (2in) piece of fresh root ginger, peeled and grated

2 tbsp olive oil

Juice of 1 lemon

100g (3½oz) feta, crumbled

70g (2¾oz) baby spinach leaves

Place the bouillon powder in a pan with about 7.5cm (3in) of water, bring to the boil, add the broccoli and simmer for 3 minutes. Add the peas and cook for a further 2 minutes, until the broccoli is just tender and the peas are completely heated through. Drain and set aside.

Place the yellow pepper, spring onion (scallion), cucumber and ginger in a bowl, add the olive oil and lemon juice and stir thoroughly, making sure the ginger is evenly mixed in. Add the broccoli, peas, feta and spinach and toss gently to combine.

This can be thrown together in a nanosecond and is a perfectly balanced meal. It also makes a lovely side dish – with or without the feta, depending on the dish you are serving it with.

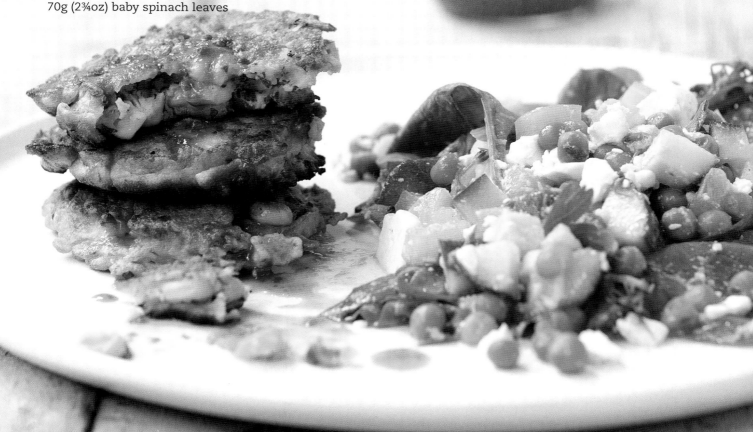

Spicy Tofu Skewers with a Chilli Pesto Dip

serves 2

1 red onion, chopped

75g (3oz) butternut squash, chopped

1 fennel bulb, chopped

2 tbsp olive oil, plus extra for sautéing

½ tsp harissa

200g (7oz) tofu, cubed

Tofu loves to soak up flavours... With this easy recipe you can serve an impressively fancy dish very quickly, and the dip is just delectable!

First, make the dip (see below). Next, preheat the oven to 180°C/350°F/gas mark 4.

Toss the chopped vegetables in 1 tablespoon of the olive oil, then place on a baking tray (cookie sheet) and bake for 35–40 minutes.

Meanwhile, mix the harissa with the remaining olive oil in a bowl and toss the tofu cubes in the mixture. Heat a frying pan, add the tofu cubes and cook for 6 minutes, turning frequently.

Thread the tofu cubes and roasted vegetables onto wooden skewers and serve at once, with the dip and Mint-and-Mango-Marinated Courgette Spaghetti (see page 126).

Chilli Pesto Dip

40g (1½oz) rocket (arugula) leaves

5g (¼oz) dill

50g (2oz/⅓ cup) raw cashews

30g (1¼oz) feta

Juice ½ lemon

½ tsp ground ginger

1 small red chilli

15g (½oz/1½ heaped tbsp) raw sunflower seeds

1 tbsp olive oil

2 tbsp water

Place all the ingredients in a blender and whizz until beautifully smooth.

NUTRITIONAL NUGGET
The bright colours of all squashes and pumpkins pack a carotene-rich punch – generally speaking, the richer the colour, the higher the concentration of carotenes, which protect against heart disease. What's more, they are an excellent source of folic acid, which is important during early pregnancy, and vitamins B1, B6 and C.

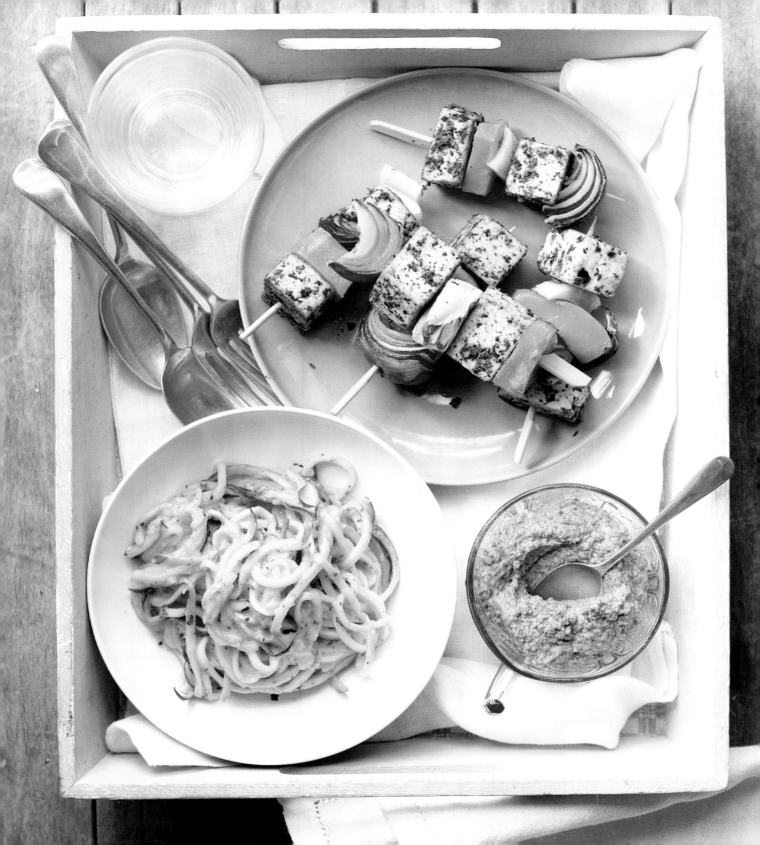

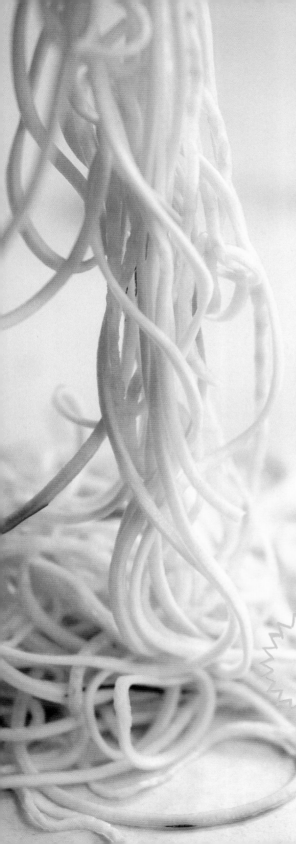

Mint-and-Mango-Marinated Courgette Spaghetti

If you fancy some pasta while you're eating the Honestly Healthy way, then this fruity dish is definitely worth a try. This is our raw 'spaghetti', and it gets everyone's head spinning at a dinner party.

serves 2

For the marinade

1 mango
4 tbsp olive oil (or more if liked)
15 mint leaves
½ tsp ground cumin
1 tsp lime juice

2.5cm (1in) piece of red chilli
5cm (2in) piece of fresh root ginger

2 courgettes (zucchini), sliced lengthways into julienne or put through a spiraliser

Peel and remove the stone from the mango. Tip the mango flesh along with all the other marinade ingredients into a blender and blend till smooth.

Pour the minty marinade over the courgette (zucchini) 'spaghetti' and work it in by hand. And that's it, ready to serve.

NUTRITIONAL NUGGET
Mangoes are a rich source of all sorts of phytochemicals – carotenoids, flavonoids and antioxidants – as well as vitamin C and fibre. These plant-based chemicals protect against heart disease and stroke, and prevent certain types of cancer. Mangoes also contain enzymes that help to improve digestion. Digestive function is further enhanced by the fresh mint in this vibrant spicy marinade.

Tomato and Mushroom Dhal

serves 4

2 tbsp olive oil
1 onion, chopped
2 garlic cloves, diced
½ tsp dried parsley
¼ tsp dried coriander (cilantro)
¼ tsp cumin seeds
200g (7oz) baby vine tomatoes
2 portobello mushrooms, sliced
900ml (1½ pints/3⅔ cups) water
400g (13oz/2 cups) split red lentils
5cm (2in) piece of red chilli, finely diced
100g (3½oz) fresh coriander (cilantro), roughly chopped
30g (1¼oz) parsley, roughly chopped
70g (2¾oz) spinach (optional)

When travelling in India I was living off dhal and when I returned home I wanted to make sure I could still get my fix! This weekday staple is such a rich source of protein and is also very comforting.

Heat the olive oil in a large pan over a medium heat and sauté the onion and garlic for 2 minutes or so, until they start to absorb the oil.

Stir in the dried parsley and coriander (cilantro), cumin seeds, tomatoes and mushrooms with 25ml (1fl oz) of the water. Allow to sweat until the tomatoes start to split and the water is absorbed.

Stir in the lentils, chilli and 400ml (14fl oz/1⅔ cups) of the remaining water and cook over a medium heat for 25–30 minutes, adding the remaining water a little at a time as necessary until the lentils are cooked and reduced to a mushy consistency but still hold their shape.

To serve, stir in the fresh coriander (cilantro) and parsley and the spinach, if using.

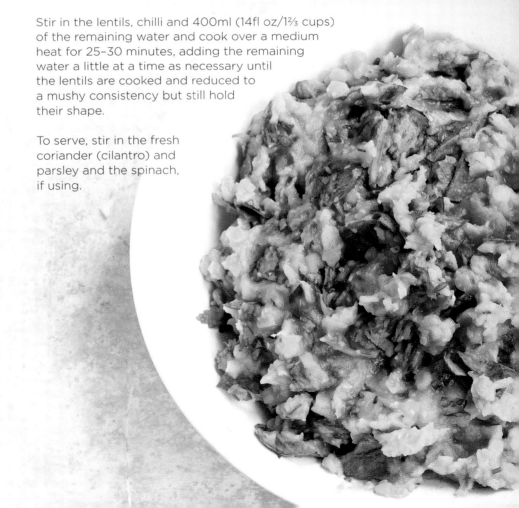

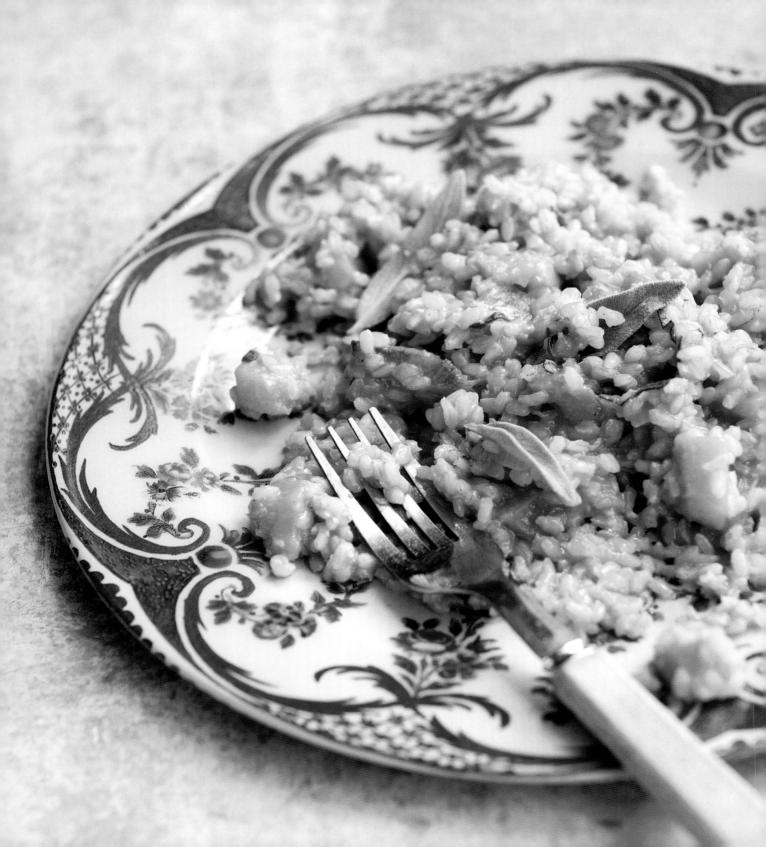

Butternut Squash Risotto

serves 4

200g (7oz) butternut squash, diced

3 tbsp olive oil

1 red onion, chopped

2 garlic cloves, chopped

180g (6oz/scant 1 cup) brown risotto rice

600ml (1 pint/2½ cups) hot vegetable stock made with 1 tbsp bouillon powder

1 handful of sage leaves, chopped, plus whole leaves to garnish

Pinch of Himalayan pink salt

Remember to stir stir stir this risotto, as that is what will make it super-creamy and rich. The stirring of the dish is almost therapeutic and meditative after a busy day, and it's well worth the time and effort.

Preheat the oven to 180°C/350°F/gas mark 4.

Place the diced butternut squash on a baking tray (cookie sheet), drizzle with 2 tablespoons of the olive oil and bake for 15 minutes, until nearly tender.

Heat the remaining olive oil in a wide-bottomed pan over a medium heat, add the onion and garlic and cook for 2–3 minutes, until softened. Add the rice and cook, stirring constantly, for 1 minute to coat the rice in oil, then reduce the heat and stir in 2 large ladlefuls of stock. Simmer, stirring gently, over a low heat until the rice has absorbed the stock, then continue adding the stock a ladleful at a time and stirring gently until it is absorbed before adding another ladleful.

After 30 minutes stir in the butternut squash and the chopped sage leaves, then continue to add the stock until the rice is cooked but al dente – this will take about 50 minutes. Season with a pinch of salt.

Serve at once, garnished with whole sage leaves.

TIP
Once you have become familiar with how to make this dish, try replacing the butternut squash with other vegetables for a different flavour or texture. Remember that the harder the vegetable, the longer you need to cook it, and vice versa for softer veg – if you are using mushrooms, for instance, you only need to throw them in at the end.

Red Rice and Beetroot Risotto

serves 4

2 tbsp olive oil

1 red onion, chopped

2 garlic cloves, chopped

180g (6oz/scant 1 cup)
   Camargue red rice

600ml (1 pint/2½ cups) hot
   vegetable stock, made with
   1 tbsp bouillon powder

160g (5½oz) beetroot (beet), cut
   into chunks

1 handful of parsley, chopped

100g (3½oz) feta

This might take a little more time than a normal risotto but my oh my, doesn't it taste delicious? The vibrancy of the red rice along with the juice from the beetroot (beet) makes this dish look so beautiful.

Heat the olive oil in a wide-bottomed pan over a medium heat, add the onion and garlic and cook for 2–3 minutes, until softened.

Add the rice and cook, stirring constantly, for 1 minute to coat the rice in oil, then reduce the heat and stir in 2 large ladlefuls of stock. Simmer, stirring gently, over a low heat until the rice has absorbed the stock, then continue adding the stock a ladleful at a time and stirring gently until it is absorbed before adding another ladleful.

After 10 minutes of cooking, add the beetroot (beet) chunks. After 25 minutes, add most of the chopped parsley, then continue to add the stock until the rice is cooked but al dente – this will take 30–40 minutes. At the last minute, stir in most of the feta to make the risotto wonderfully creamy.

Serve garnished with the remaining feta and chopped parsley.

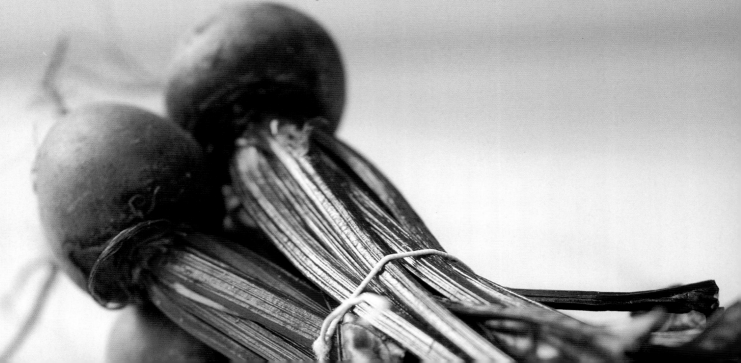

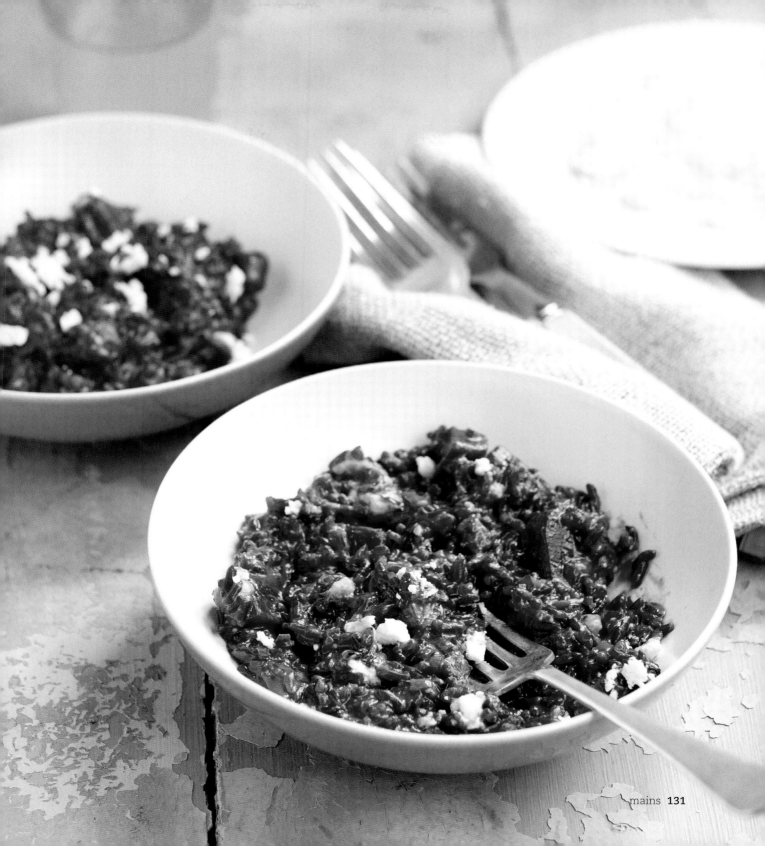

Pea Carbonara

serves 2

3 tbsp olive oil

1 shallot, diced

2 small garlic cloves,
   thinly sliced

225g (7½oz/scant 2 cups)
   frozen peas, defrosted and
   drained

100g (3½oz) broad (fava) beans
   (fresh, shelled or frozen,
   defrosted and drained)

Himalayan pink salt

Freshly ground black pepper

180g (6oz) gluten-free spaghetti

2 egg yolks

80g (3oz) goat's Cheddar, grated

Leaves from 2 large handfuls of
   fresh mint, half chopped and
   half left whole

1 red chilli, sliced diagonally, to
   garnish (optional)

Who says you can't indulge in a yummy bowl of creamy pasta? I was not prepared to give up this wonderful dish from my childhood – so we found a way to make it the Honestly Healthy way!

Heat the olive oil in a pan and sauté the shallots, garlic, peas and broad (fava) beans over a medium heat, partially covered, until the shallots are soft. Season to taste with salt and pepper.

Meanwhile, bring a large pan of salted water to the boil and add the spaghetti. Cook according to the packet instructions, then drain well.

In a bowl, mix the egg yolks with half the goat's cheese and the chopped mint and season with black pepper.

Using tongs, transfer the cooked, drained spaghetti to the pan with the shallot mixture. Pour in the egg mixture, turning the spaghetti into the mixture with the tongs over a very low heat to coat the pasta and thicken the egg mixture.

Serve sprinkled with the remaining grated cheese and garnished with chilli slices, if you like, and whole mint leaves.

TIP
Wheat-free pasta tends to disintegrate quite easily so be gentle when coating it with the sauce.

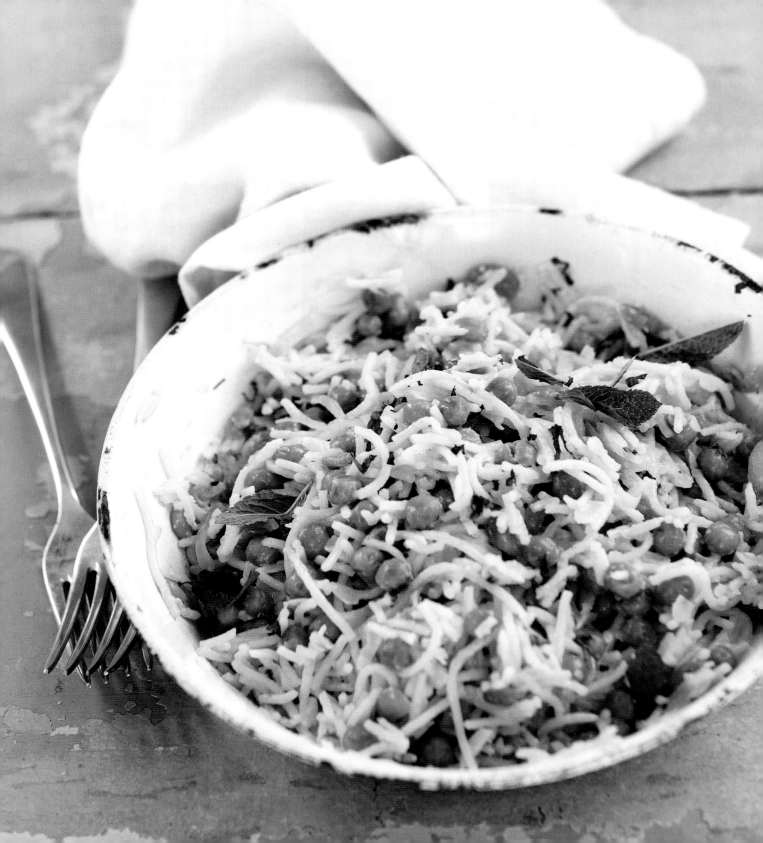

Spicy Bean Burgers with Cajun Wedges and Superslaw

serves 4

1½ tbsp olive oil

1 tsp ground coriander

1 tsp turmeric

2 fat garlic cloves, chopped

1 small red chilli, chopped

75g (3oz) onion, chopped

60g (2½oz) carrot, grated

60g (2½oz) courgette (zucchini), grated

50g (2oz/scant ⅓ cup) fresh or frozen sweetcorn kernels

250g (8oz/1¼ cups) canned black-eyed beans, rinsed and drained

250g (8oz/1¼ cups) canned black beans, rinsed and drained

1 tsp Himalayan pink salt

1 tbsp chopped fresh coriander (cilantro)

50g (2oz/¼ cup) millet flakes

Polenta (cornmeal), for coating

Sunflower oil, for sautéing

To serve

Cajun Sweet Potato Wedges (see page 136)

Superslaw (see page 136)

There's nothing better than sinking your teeth into a (healthy) burger and indulging in some home-made spicy potato wedges and slaw, to boot.

Heat the oil in a large saucepan, add the ground coriander and turmeric and sauté for 2 minutes, then add the garlic and chilli and sauté for 1–2 minutes, until softened. Add the onion and sauté for a further 3–4 minutes to soften the onion, adding a splash of water if the mixture gets too dry.

Add the grated carrot and courgette (zucchini) and sauté for 1–2 minutes, until softened. Add the sweetcorn kernels and sauté for 2 minutes, until softened. Add the beans and sauté for a further 2 minutes, until softened. Stir in the salt.

Transfer the ingredients to a mixing bowl and stir in the chopped coriander (cilantro) and millet flakes. When cool enough to handle, form the mixture into 8 burgers, kneading the mixture lightly to break down the beans.

Spread a generous layer of polenta (cornmeal) on a plate and coat the burgers well, then chill in the refrigerator for 30 minutes.

Meanwhile, preheat the oven to 160°C/325°F/gas mark 3.

Heat a little sunflower oil in a frying pan and, working in batches, cook the burgers for about 2 minutes on each side, until golden. Transfer to a baking tray (cookie sheet) lined with baking parchment and bake for 20 minutes, until cooked through.

Serve hot alongside Cajun Sweet Potato Wedges and Superslaw.

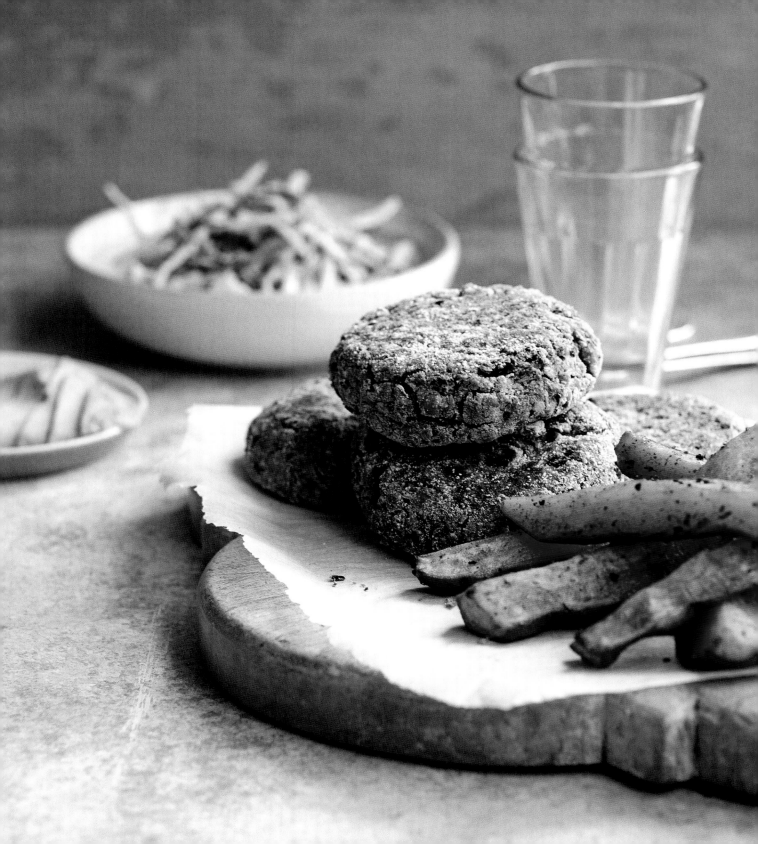

Cajun Sweet Potato Wedges

serves 4

3 sweet potatoes, peeled and
cut into large wedges
2 tbsp olive oil
Cajun spice mix, to taste

Place the sweet potato wedges in
a large bowl with the olive oil and
Cajun spice mix, to taste, and toss
well to coat thoroughly. Transfer
to a baking tray (cookie sheet)
and cook in a preheated oven,
160°C/325°F/gas mark 3, for
30 minutes, or until golden brown.

No need to feel guilty
with these – they are
far healthier than
chip-shop offerings.

Superslaw

serves 4

65g (2½oz) red cabbage, finely
sliced
150g (5oz) white cabbage, finely
sliced
50g (2oz) sweet potato, grated
50g (2oz) celeriac, grated
50g (2oz) apple, grated
25g (1oz) spring onion
(scallion), finely sliced
25g (1oz/generous ⅛ cup) raw
sunflower seeds, soaked for
30 minutes and drained
1 tsp Himalayan pink salt
Ground black pepper

Tahini/cashew mayo
1 heaped tbsp tahini
1 heaped tsp cashew butter
1 tbsp olive oil
Juice of ½ lime
½ tsp white miso
2 garlic cloves
Himalayan pink salt
Freshly ground pepper

To make the tahini/cashew mayo,
whizz all the ingredients in a blender,
gradually adding as much water as
necessary to make a smooth sauce.
Season with salt and pepper, to taste.

Combine the coleslaw ingredients in
a large bowl. Pour over the mayo and,
using your hands, massage together
until all the coleslaw ingredients are
well coated with the mayo.

Why not make up a big
batch of the 'mayo' –
you can store it in the
fridge for up to five
days and use it as a
creamy salad dressing.

WHAT IS WHITE MISO?
Great for light dishes, white miso is fermented
for only 2–8 weeks, unlike all other misos. It has a
creamy texture and is fantastic for salad dressings.

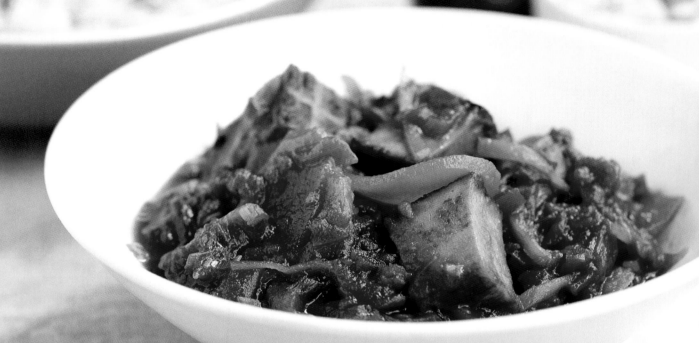

100g (3½oz) carrots

1 tbsp soya bean paste

300ml (½ pint/scant 1¼ cups)
    boiling water

100g (3½oz) fresh root ginger,
    thinly sliced

1 lemongrass stalk, peeled and
    finely chopped

10 plum tomatoes, diced

½ green pepper, diced

½ red pepper, diced

50g (2oz) edamame beans

½ onion, thinly sliced

1 tsp tamari

1 tbsp honey

150g (5oz) smoked tofu, cubed

Cooked brown rice, to serve

Toasted cashews, to garnish

Sweet and Sour Tofu

I have always wanted to find an alternative to this
classic Chinese dish as I do enjoy the taste, but
obviously wanted something that was healthier –
and I am so glad I have.

Thinly slice the carrots on the diagonal and blanch in a pan of boiling
water for 1 minute.

In a separate pan, dissolve the soya bean paste in the measured
amount of boiling water, then add the ginger and lemongrass. Bring
the mixture to the boil, then simmer for 25–30 minutes, until reduced
and infused with flavour.

Add the diced tomatoes and cook for about 5 minutes, until reduced.
Add the peppers, edamame beans and onion and cook for 3 minutes.
Stir in the tamari and honey, then add the tofu and heat through.

Serve with rice, garnished with toasted cashews.

Chickpea and Sweet Potato Stew

serves 4

2 tbsp olive oil

1 red onion, finely sliced

2 garlic cloves, finely sliced

600ml (1 pint/2½ cups) water

1 sweet potato, cut into 2.5cm
(1in) cubes

5 large vine tomatoes, cut into
quarters

3 fresh or dried bay leaves

½ red chilli, finely chopped

1 tsp ground cumin

Pinch of cayenne pepper

1 small aubergine (eggplant),
quartered lengthways and
cut into 1cm (½in) slices

800g (1lb 10oz/4 cups) canned
chickpeas, rinsed and
drained

Coriander (cilantro), roughly
chopped, to serve

Cooked brown rice, to serve
(optional)

I leave the skin on the sweet potato as it contains so many nutrients and is very tasty – just make sure you scrub well before cooking. Vine tomatoes are very tasty but you can use plum or beef tomatoes instead. This is a perfect cosy lunch or dinner on a cold day.

Heat the olive oil in a large pan over a medium heat, stir in the onion and garlic and cook for 3–4 minutes, until softened. Add 50ml (2fl oz/scant ¼ cup) of the water and stir in the sweet potato, then crush the chopped tomatoes into the pan and add the bay leaves. Cook for 5 minutes.

Add the chilli, cumin, cayenne and 300ml (½ pint/scant 1¼ cups) of the water and simmer for 15 minutes, or until reduced to a thick sauce. Add the aubergine (eggplant), chickpeas and remaining water and simmer for a further 10 minutes, stirring frequently, until the aubergine (eggplant) is tender and the sauce is reduced.

Serve the stew, sprinkled with some chopped coriander (cilantro), on its own or with brown rice.

NUTRITIONAL NUGGET
Did you know that cayenne pepper helps you to lose weight because of its thermogenic properties, which raise metabolism?

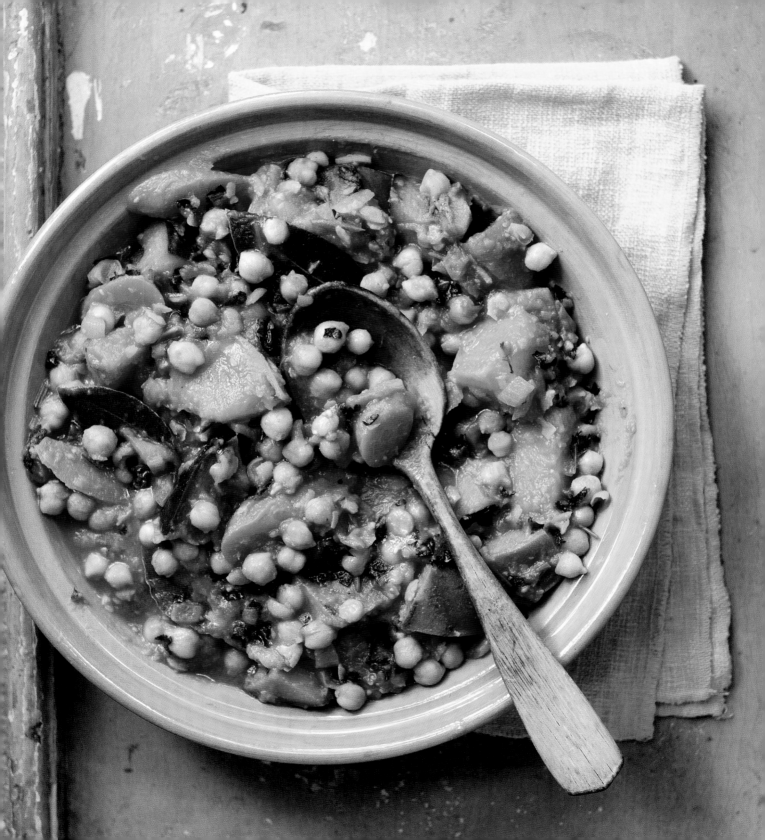

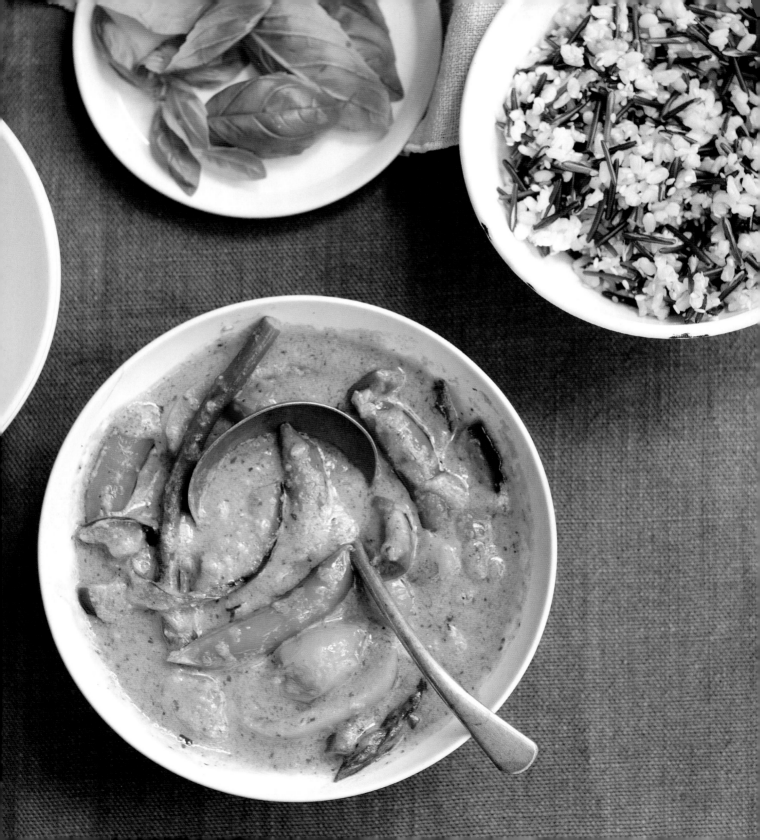

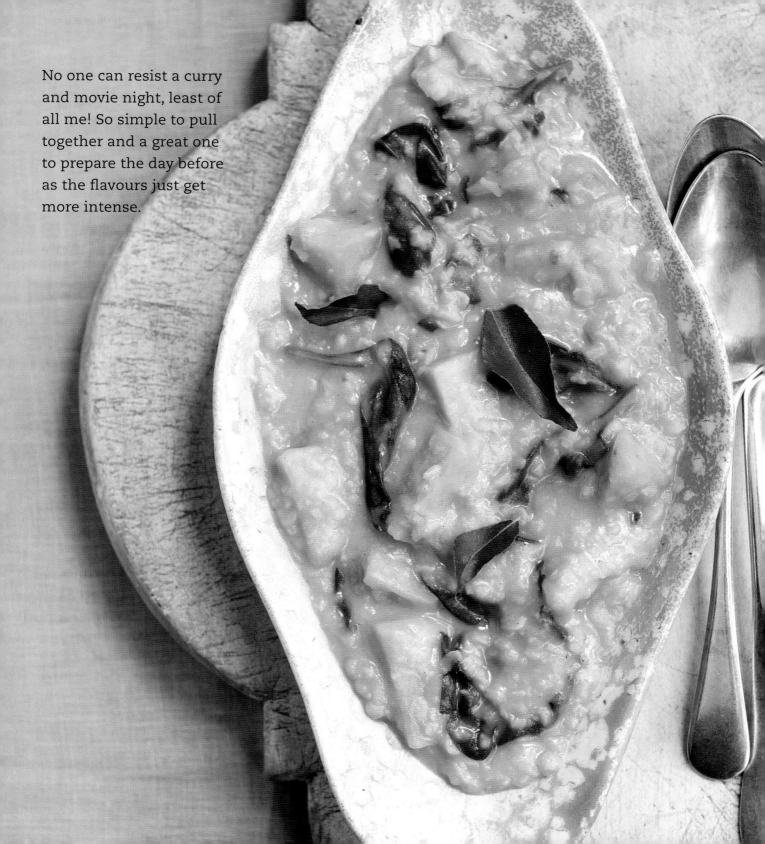

No one can resist a curry and movie night, least of all me! So simple to pull together and a great one to prepare the day before as the flavours just get more intense.

Thai Yellow Curry with Jasmine Brown Rice

serves 2

For the curry paste
3 shallots, chopped
1 lemongrass stalk, peeled and chopped
2 small red chillies, deseeded
5 garlic cloves
½ handful of coriander (cilantro)
5cm (2in) piece of galangal, peeled and chopped
1 fresh or dried kaffir lime leaf
1 tbsp ground coriander seeds
1½ tbsp mild chilli powder
½ tsp turmeric
2 tsp rice syrup
¼ tsp Himalayan pink salt

For the curry
1 lemongrass stalk
1 tbsp coconut oil
5 heaped tsp curry paste
75g (3oz) aubergine (eggplant)
400ml (14fl oz/1⅔ cups) coconut milk
60g (2½oz) yellow pepper
45g (1¾oz) sugar snap peas
50g (2oz) fine Thai asparagus
65g (2½oz) red and yellow cherry tomatoes, halved
150ml (¼ pint/⅔ cup) water
4 Thai basil leaves, shredded
Tamari, to taste

(Pictured on page 140.) If you have never made a curry paste from scratch, this is the easiest one to start with. It's worth the effort and makes you feel like a culinary genius! Serve with jasmine brown rice for authenticity.

To make the paste, whizz all the ingredients in a blender until smooth.

Next, make the curry. Peel and bash the lemongrass and chop into pieces. Heat the coconut oil and sauté the lemongrass over a low heat for 2 minutes to infuse the oil. Add the curry paste and sauté for 2 minutes.

Halve the aubergine (eggplant) lengthways and thinly slice and simmer in 200ml (7fl oz/generous ¾ cup) of the coconut milk for 5 minutes. Cut the pepper into strips and pop that in the pan and simmer for a further 5 minutes.

Add the sugar snap peas, asparagus and tomatoes, the remaining coconut milk and as much water as required to make the consistency you like and cook for 4–5 minutes, until the vegetables are just tender. Stir in the basil and a splash of tamari, to taste.

I like this curry served with some jasmine brown rice sprinkled with toasted sesame seeds and grated lime zest.

TIP
Take care not to overheat the oil and burn the spices, as this will distort the wondrous flavour of the curry.

Mung Bean Curry

serves 4

½ tsp coconut oil
1 red onion, chopped
1 tsp finely chopped garlic
   cloves
1 tsp grated fresh root ginger
3–4 small red or green chillies,
   finely chopped
1 heaped tsp soya bean paste
1 tsp cinnamon
1½ tsp turmeric
1 tsp paprika
2 fresh or dried kaffir lime
   leaves
3 plum tomatoes, chopped
1 sweet potato, diced
400ml (14fl oz/1⅔ cups)
   coconut milk
150g (5oz/generous ⅔ cup) split
   mung beans, soaked for 1
   hour and cooked
1 handful of baby spinach
   leaves (optional)
Coriander (cilantro),
   chopped, to garnish
Brown rice, to serve

(Pictured on page 141.) No need for an introduction to this one. Everyone loves this dish, even children, as it's so warming and comforting but leaves you feeling light.

Heat the coconut oil in a large pan, then wipe the pan with a piece of kitchen paper (paper towel). Add the onion, garlic, ginger, chillies and soya bean paste and sauté for 2–3 minutes to soften the onion.

Add the spices, lime leaves and tomatoes and cook for a further 2–3 minutes to soften the tomatoes. Add the sweet potato and cook for 3 minutes, then add the coconut milk and mung beans. Simmer for 15–20 minutes, until the sweet potato is tender.

Adding a handful of spinach at the end is a nice touch or just add chopped coriander (cilantro) as a garnish. Serve with brown rice.

NUTRITIONAL NUGGET
The mung bean has one of the widest ranges of nutrients of any bean or pulse and is as versatile in its uses. This is a real energy food.

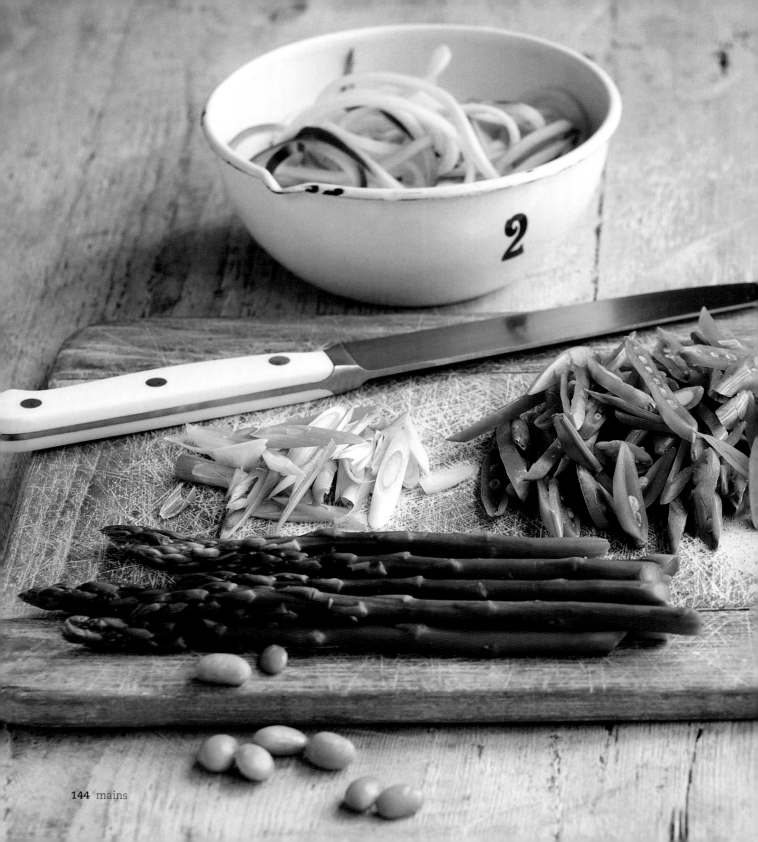

Raw Pad Thai

serves 2

♥ ♥ ♥ ⚭

2 courgettes (zucchini)
1 carrot
20g (¾oz) edamame beans
50g (2oz) mangetout (snow
  peas), thinly sliced diagonally
50g (2oz) fine asparagus, thinly
  sliced diagonally

For the sauce

45g (1¾oz/scant ⅓ cup) raw
  cashews, soaked for 2 hours
3 fresh or dried dates
1 lemongrass stalk, peeled
  and chopped
10g (½oz) fresh root ginger,
  chopped
2 fat garlic cloves
Grated zest and juice of 1 lime
1 tbsp tamari
1 tsp dried chilli flakes

To garnish

1 tbsp finely chopped coriander
  (cilantro)
Lightly toasted cashews
1 spring onion (scallion), thinly
  sliced diagonally

This is such a fun one to prepare, especially if you have kids, as the spiraliser is a great implement to play with. Of course, the grown-ups enjoy it too.

To make the sauce, drain the cashews and then whizz all the ingredients in a blender, gradually adding water until smooth.

Spiralise the courgettes (zucchini) and carrot to make thin noodles and place in a bowl. Add the edamame beans, mangetout (snow peas) and asparagus. Pour over the sauce and mix to coat the vegetables evenly.

Serve garnished with chopped coriander (cilantro), cashews and spring onion (scallion).

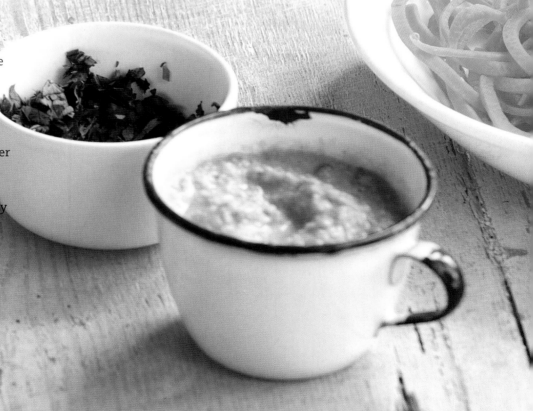

Aubergine with Cashew Pesto

serves 2

1 aubergine (eggplant), halved
  lengthways
4 tbsp olive oil
50g (2oz/⅓ cup) raw cashews
40g (1½oz) coriander (cilantro)
1 garlic clove
50g (2oz) feta, crumbled

This simple but tasty bake takes no effort whatsoever and (although meatless) is a meaty and complete meal, with the cashews adding great protein to this dish.

Preheat the oven to 170°C/340°F/gas mark 3½.

Place the aubergine (eggplant) halves cut-side up on a baking tray (cookie sheet), drizzle with 2 tablespoons of the olive oil and bake for about 25 minutes, until almost tender.

Meanwhile, whizz the cashews, coriander (cilantro), garlic and remaining olive oil in a blender to a rough paste. When the aubergine (eggplant) halves are almost tender, coat them with the pesto and return to the oven for a further 10 minutes, until the pesto starts to crisp and brown.

Serve sprinkled with feta and accompanied with Sweet Tomato Tabbouleh (see below).

Sweet Tomato Tabbouleh

serves 2

80g (3oz) baby vine tomatoes,
  deseeded, diced and drained
100g (3½oz) flat-leaf parsley,
  roughly chopped
30g (1¼oz/scant ¼ cup) raw
  sesame seeds
2 tbsp olive oil
Juice of 2 lemons
2 tsp agave syrup

Place the diced tomatoes in a bowl and stir in the parsley and sesame seeds. Whisk together the remaining ingredients and drizzle onto the tomato mixture and toss together.

NUTRITIONAL NUGGET
Parsley is very high in iron to keep you going all day.

This refreshing, zingy salad is honestly one of my favourites – I could sit and eat a whole bowlful without getting bored! The sesame seeds are a rich source of minerals, including calcium and selenium.

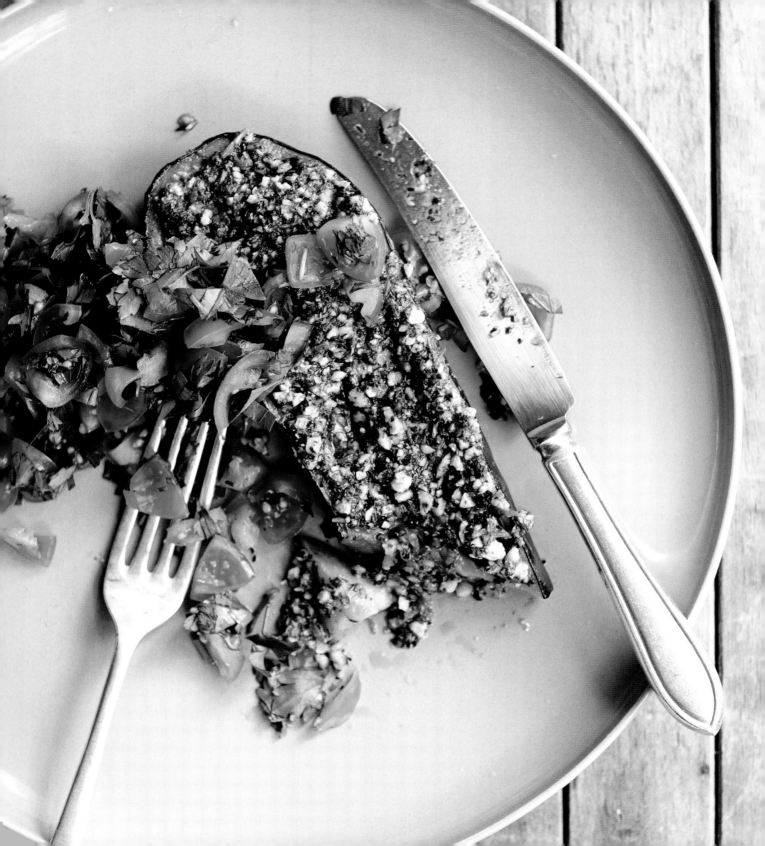

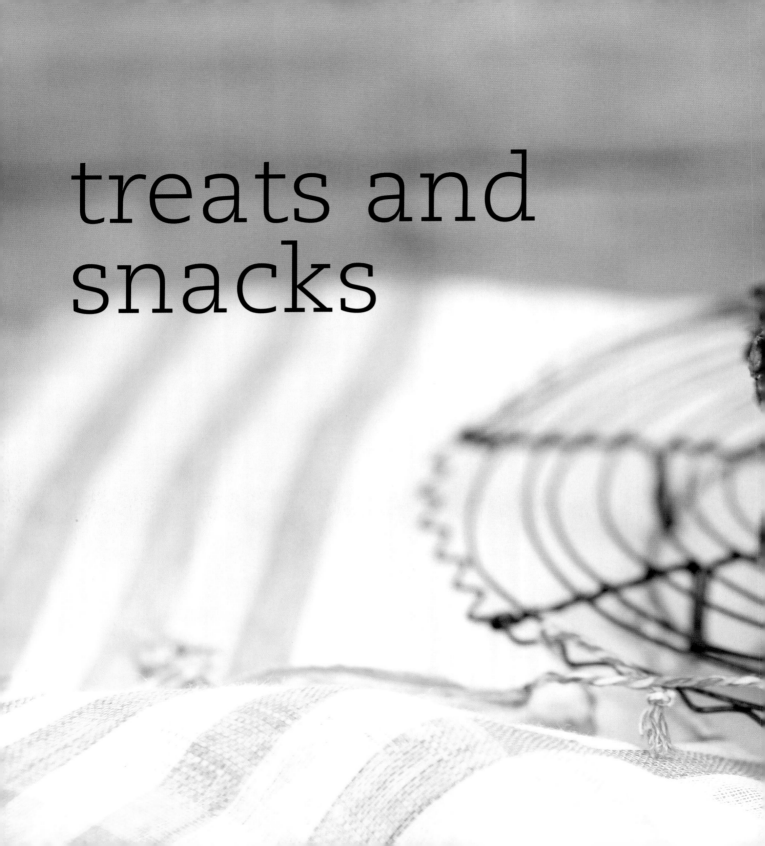

treats and snacks

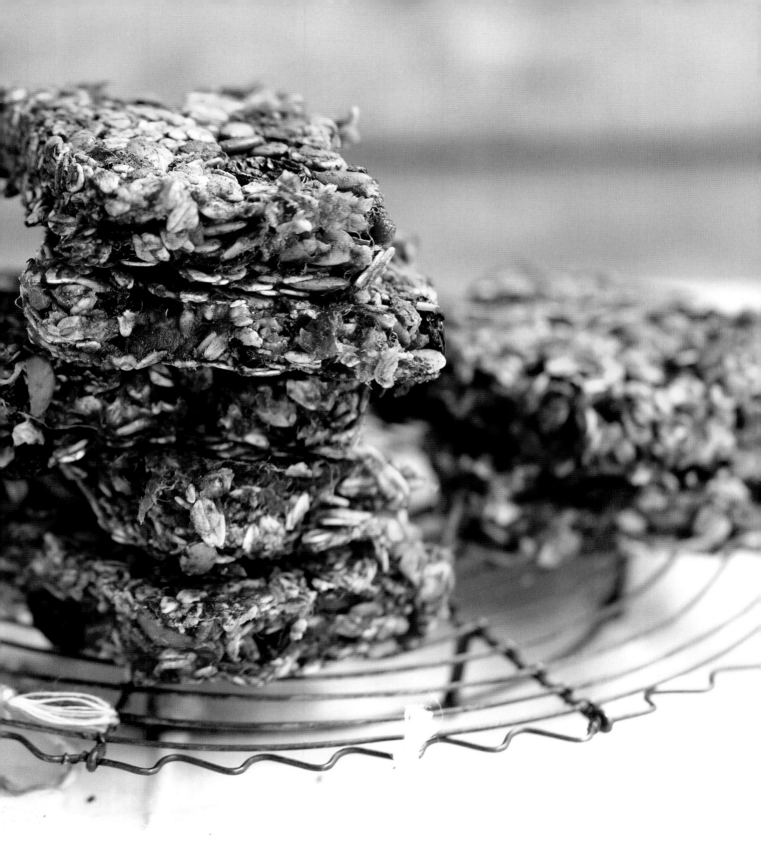

Granola Bars

makes 12

200g (7oz/scant 2¼ cups)
   jumbo rolled oats
200g (7oz/generous 1⅛ cups)
   dried dates, chopped
100g (3½oz) dried figs, chopped
75g (3oz/scant ⅔ cup) goji
   berries
75g (3oz/scant ½ cup) dried
   blueberries
75g (3oz/scant ½ cup) raisins
2 tbsp raw flax seeds
Pinch of cinnamon
½ tsp vanilla extract
½ tbsp lúcuma powder
1 tbsp maca powder
2 tbsp raw pumpkin seeds
1 tbsp agave syrup

NUTRITIONAL NUGGET
Nothing beats your own
granola bars for ensuring
additive-free, B-vitamin-rich,
high-energy snack bars.

(Pictured on pages 148–149.) These perfect guilt-free snacks are full of nutrient-dense superfoods (goji berries, lúcuma and maca powder, blueberries and agave syrup), which are rich in antioxidants and so help to heal and feed your body, giving you more energy and great health. Everyone loves these and can't quite believe that they taste so great and are so good for you. Leave them to cool completely before demolishing!

Preheat the oven to 150°C/300°F/gas mark 2.

Spread the oats on a large baking tray (cookie sheet) and bake for about 20 minutes, or until golden brown, turning them over every 5 minutes or so. Remove from the oven and leave to cool in the tray.

Place the dates and figs in a pan and cover with water to double the depth. Bring to the boil, then simmer for about 45 minutes, stirring occasionally and adding extra water if the mixture gets too dry. This is going to be your syrup, so you want to reduce the dates and figs to a sloppy, sweet liquid. The cooking time will depend on how dry the fruit is – the drier it is, the longer it will take. Once the mixture has turned into a syrup, take the pan off the heat.

Add the goji berries, blueberries, raisins and flax seeds, and leave the mixture to rest for 10 minutes to let the berries and raisins swell and absorb some of the syrup.

Stir in the cinnamon, vanilla extract, lúcuma, maca, pumpkin seeds and agave syrup. Add the oats, a little at a time, stirring after each addition to make sure they are completely coated in the syrup.

Spread the sweet oaty mixture evenly in a large rectangular baking tray (cookie sheet), to a thickness of about 1.5cm (¾in). Bake for 15–20 minutes, until lovely and golden.

Remove the granola from the oven and cut it into 12 squares. As soon as they are cool enough to handle, carefully transfer them to a wire rack, placing them upside down, and leave to cool completely.

Chocolate Peanut Butter Cups

makes 6

100g (3½oz/½ cup) raw cacao butter

4 tbsp agave syrup

75g (3oz/¾ cup) raw cacao powder

150g (5oz/1 cup) unsalted peanuts

2 tbsp coconut oil

1 tsp nutritional yeast flakes

I grew up on Reese's peanut butter cups so recreating this far healthier option was like taking a trip down memory lane for my taste buds!

Place the cacao butter and agave syrup in a Vitamix or high-speed blender and blend on high speed until liquid, then add the cacao powder and blend again to combine. Transfer to a bowl, then coat the bottom and sides of 6 mini paper muffin liners with the chocolate, reserving enough to make a lid for each one. Place in the freezer for 4 minutes to set.

Meanwhile, wash and dry the blender jug and whizz the remaining ingredients to form a smooth butter. Divide the peanut butter between the chocolate cups and pour a layer of chocolate over the top. Return to the freezer for 5–10 minutes to set. Store in an airtight container in the refrigerator.

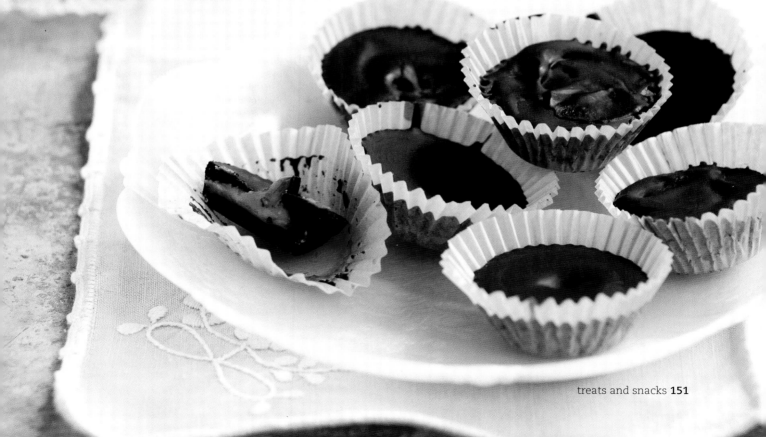

Sticky Seed Flapjacks

makes 10–12

175g (6oz/1 cup) chopped
    pitted dates
450ml (¾ pint/scant 2 cups)
    water
150g (5oz/1 cup) raw cashews
150g (5oz/1 cup) raw hazelnuts
300g (10oz/3⅓ cups) jumbo
    rolled oats
150g (5oz/scant 1 cup) raw
    pumpkin seeds
150g (5oz/scant 1 cup) raw
    sunflower seeds
475g (15oz/scant 1⅓ cups)
    agave syrup or runny honey
75g (3oz/½ cup) mixed raw
    pumpkin, sunflower and
    sesame seeds, for the
    topping

The joy of these flapjacks is that, being home-made, there are no added nasties to ruin a good intention, such as the demerara sugar used as a preservative in commercial versions. Using a range of nuts and seeds packs in the protein and provides masses of beneficial fats that feed the brain and skin and lift your mood. You'll love these.

Preheat the oven to 160°C/325°F/gas mark 3.

Place the dates and 225ml (7½fl oz/scant 1 cup) of the water in a pan, bring to the boil, then simmer until the dates are soft. Transfer to a blender, whizz to a paste and decant into a large mixing bowl.

Place the cashews and hazelnuts in the blender with the remaining water and whizz to a smooth cream. Add to the bowl with the dates.

Place the oats, pumpkin seeds and sunflower seeds in a food processor and pulse for about 1 minute, or until roughly chopped. Add these to the mixture in the bowl. Stir in the agave syrup or honey and mix thoroughly.

Transfer the mixture to a baking tray (cookie sheet) lined with baking parchment and spread out to a thickness of 1–2cm (½–¾in). Sprinkle with the mixed seeds and bake for 20 minutes, until golden.

Leave to cool in the baking tray (cookie sheet), then cut into slices.

WHAT IS AGAVE SYRUP?
Sometimes described as agave nectar, this sugar alternative is naturally extracted from the inner core of the cactus-like agave plant. Unlike refined sugar, agave syrup is absorbed slowly into the blood-stream, thereby avoiding the sugar highs and lows associated with refined sugar.

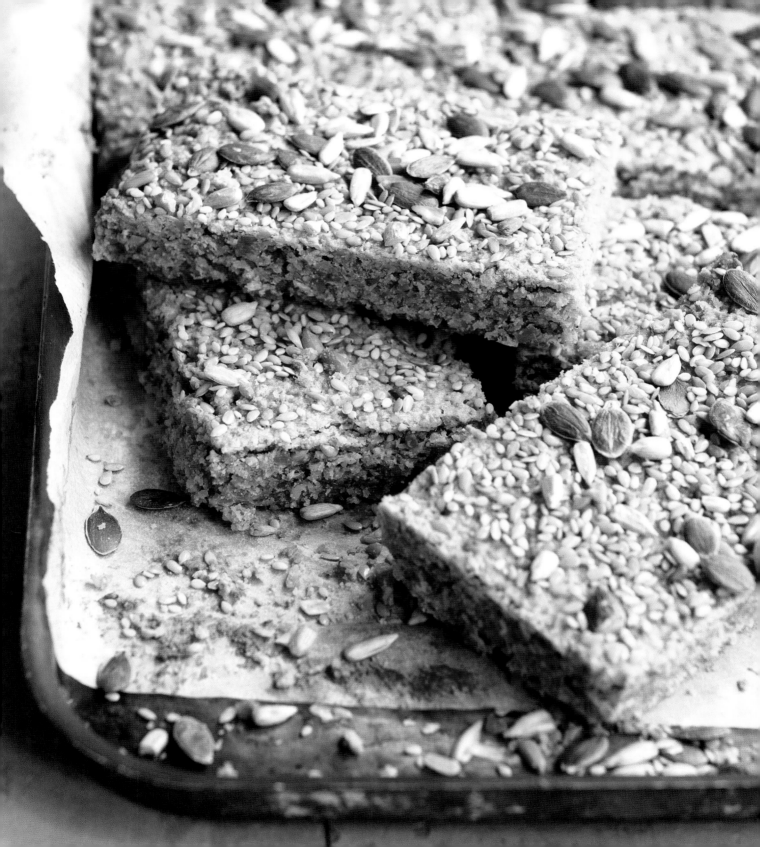

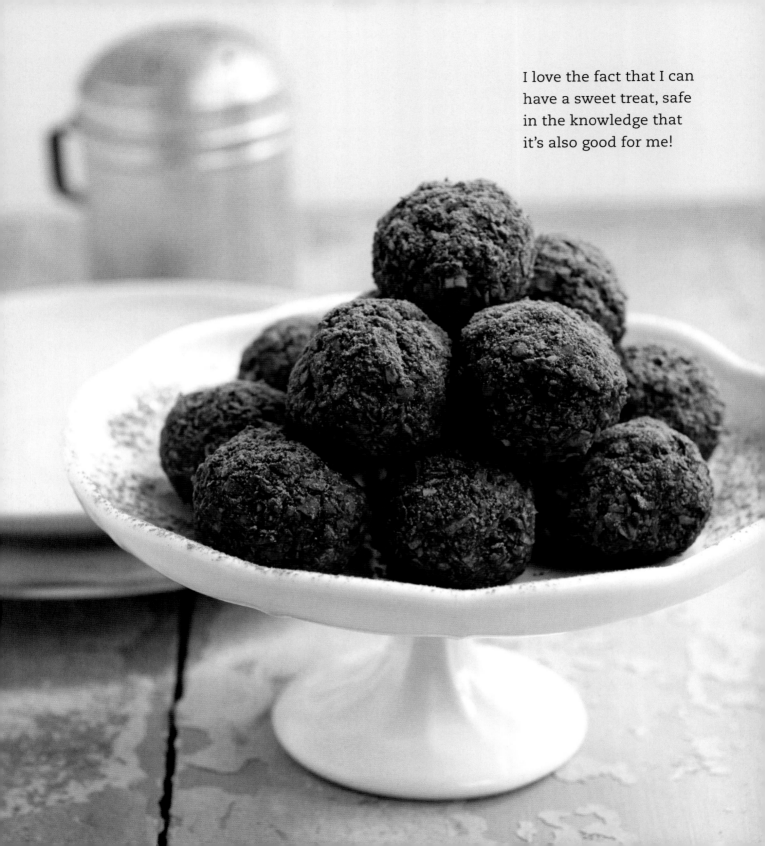

I love the fact that I can have a sweet treat, safe in the knowledge that it's also good for me!

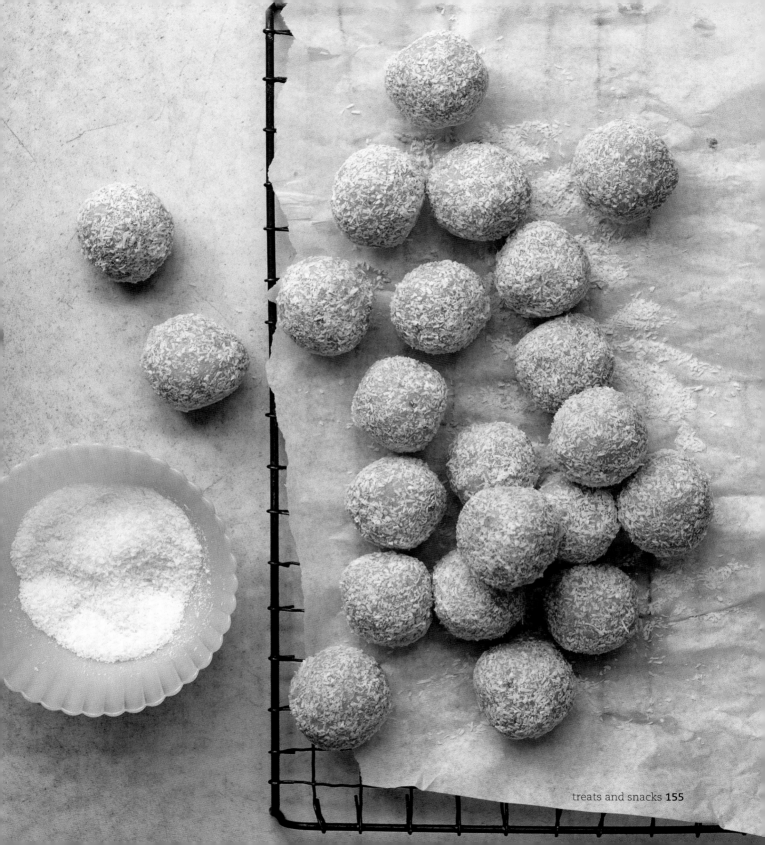

Chocolate Coconut Balls

makes 12

10 fresh dates, pitted

50g (2oz/½ cup) raw cacao
    powder

25g (1oz/generous ⅛ cup) raw
    almonds

200g (7oz/4 cups) coconut
    flakes

30g (1¼oz) agave syrup

2 tbsp coconut oil

1 tsp xylitol

2 tbsp water

(Pictured on page 154.) Who can resist a super-cute and tasty chocolate ball? Not me! If you need your choccie fix, then this one will hit the spot.

Preheat the oven to 180°C/350°F/gas mark 4.

Mix the dates, cacao powder and almonds in a blender or food processor for about 1 minute to make a sticky, chunky paste. Add the remaining ingredients and blend to a rough consistency.

Transfer the mixture to a bowl, divide it into 12 pieces and roll into balls. Place them on a baking tray (cookie sheet) lined with baking parchment and bake for 10 minutes. Then allow to cool.

Raw Mango Coconut Balls

makes 20

250g (8oz/3½ cups) desiccated
    coconut (dry unsweetened
    shredded coconut)

200g (7oz) dried unsweetened
    unsulphured mango, soaked
    in water for 30 minutes and
    drained

40g (1½oz) agave syrup

8 tbsp coconut oil

2 tsp freshly grated lemon zest

(Pictured on page 155.) For a mid-morning pick-me-up try these powerful little balls of natural sweetness – they will literally melt in your mouth.

Place 225g (7½oz/3¼ cups) of the coconut in a food processor with the mango, agave syrup, coconut oil and lemon zest and pulse until the mixture comes together. Transfer this to a bowl.

Put the remaining coconut in a separate bowl. Form the mixture into small balls and coat them in the coconut.

Freeze the coconut balls for 20 minutes on a baking tray (cookie sheet) lined with baking parchment. Store in an airtight container in the refrigerator.

Nutty Cookies

makes 15

135g (4½oz/¾ cup) raw Brazil nuts

250g (8oz/1½ cups) raw almonds

80g (3oz/scant 1⅔ cups) coconut flakes

175g (6oz/1 cup) dried prunes

85g (3¼oz/½ cup) dried apricots

30g (1¼oz/generous ⅛ cup) raw sunflower seeds

40g (1¾oz/generous ¼ cup) raw pumpkin seeds

Finely grated zest of 1 lemon

About 2 tbsp apple juice

These are surely contenders for the winners of 'the healthiest cookies in the world' competition but that doesn't mean they don't have to pack great flavour in.

Preheat the oven to 150°C/300°F/gas mark 2.

Place the ingredients in a food processor and whizz until the mixture comes together, adding a little extra apple juice if necessary.

Divide the mixture into 15 pieces and shape into balls. Place on a baking tray (cookie sheet) lined with baking parchment and flatten each ball to a thickness of 5mm (¼in).

Bake for 15 minutes, or until just firm, and then cool on a wire rack.

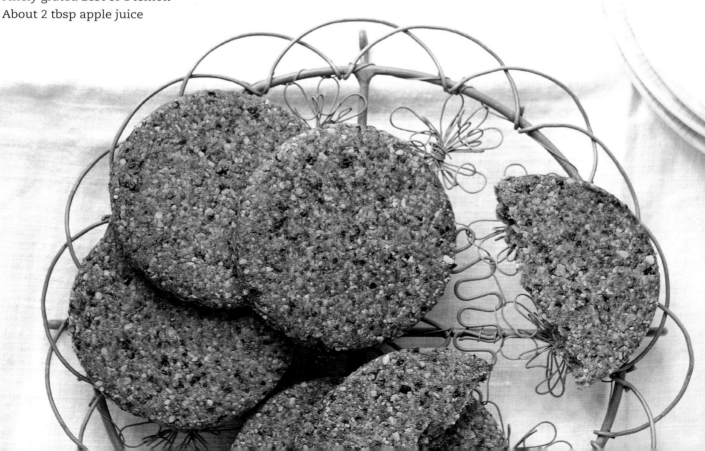

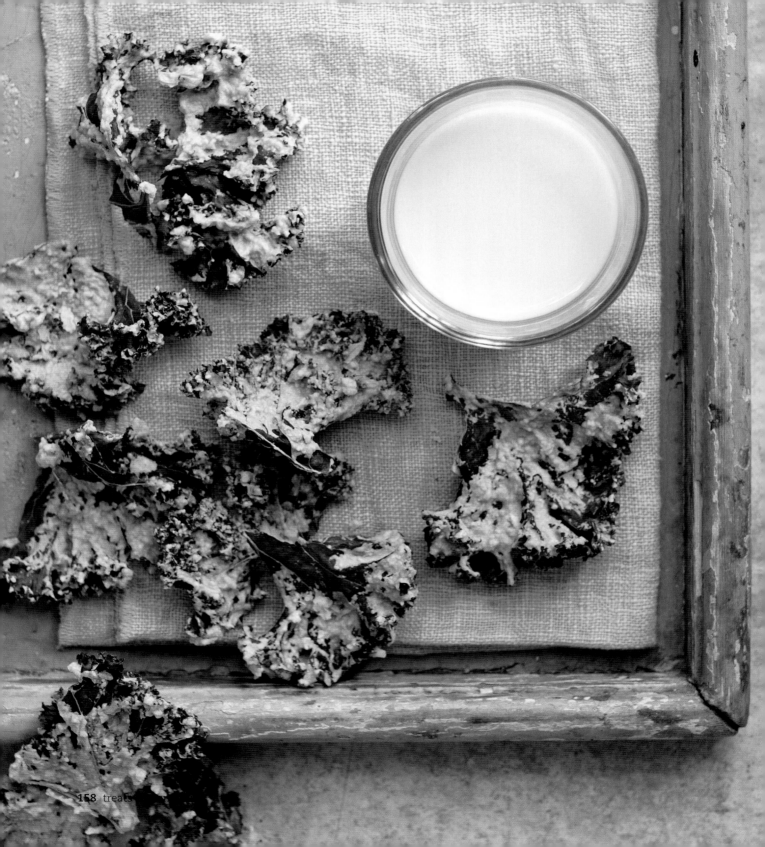

'Cheesy' Kale Chips

The first time I tried a kale chip I was simply blown away at its sheer super-tastiness. I couldn't quite believe that a dehydrated vegetable could be both quite so delicious and quite so nutritious.

makes 60g (2½oz)

♥ ♥ ⚘

6g (¼oz) thyme leaves

Juice of 1 lemon

60g (2½oz) nutritional yeast flakes

100g (3½oz/⅔ cup) raw cashews

120ml (4fl oz/½ cup) water

60g (2½oz) kale, chopped into 5cm (2in) pieces

Whizz all the ingredients, except the kale, in a blender until smooth. Pour the mixture over the kale pieces and, using your hands, coat the kale pieces gently but thoroughly.

Spread out on a dehydrator sheet and place in the dehydrator for 10 hours. (If you don't have a dehydrator, turn to page 54 for how to get the effect using an oven.)

NUTRITIONAL NUGGET
Sources of B12 are limited for vegetarians and vegans so these tasty little flakes of nutritional yeast are a great way of getting this exuberant vitamin into your life.

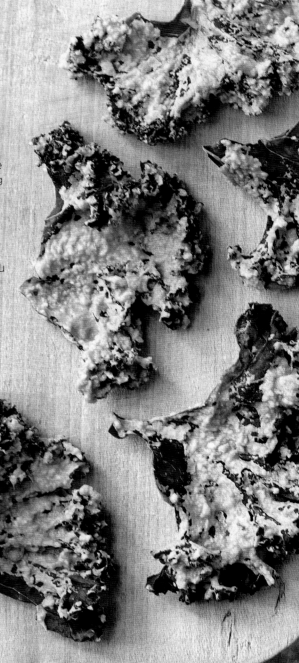

Coconut Bread

makes 1 small loaf

280g (9¼oz/2¼ cups)
   wholegrain spelt flour

2 tsp baking powder

2 tsp cinnamon

130g (4¼oz/scant 2⅔ cups)
   desiccated coconut (dry
   unsweetened shredded
   coconut)

75g (3oz/scant ⅓ cup) goat's
   butter, plus extra for greasing

150g (5oz/scant ½ cup) agave
   syrup

2 eggs

300ml (½ pint/scant 1¼ cups)
   Brown Rice Milk (see page 57)

1 tsp vanilla extract

Yes, you can have your cake and eat it, Honestly Healthy style. This wondrous coconut bread will satisfy anyone's sweet tooth and makes a perfect afternoon treat.

Preheat the oven to 180°C/350°F/gas mark 4. Grease a small loaf tin (19 x 8.5cm/7.5 x 3.5in) with goat's butter.

Sift the flour, baking powder, cinnamon and ground coconut flakes into a bowl.

In a separate bowl, cream the goat's butter with the agave syrup. Add the eggs, milk and vanilla and then stir well to combine. Add the wet ingredients to the dry ingredients and combine.

Transfer the mixture to the loaf tin and bake for about 1 hour. The loaf will rise slightly and have a golden crust. To test whether it is cooked, insert the tip of a sharp knife or a skewer into the centre of the loaf. If it comes out clean, the loaf is ready.

Leave to cool in the tin for 10 minutes, then turn out onto a wire rack to cool completely.

Nut Butter

To make any nut butter, simply blend however many nuts you need for your portion until creamy; the nut oils make it beautifully buttery.

Our favourites: almond butter and cashew butter.

TIP
When you are making your nut butter, if your blender is struggling to cream the nuts just add a few drops of olive oil.

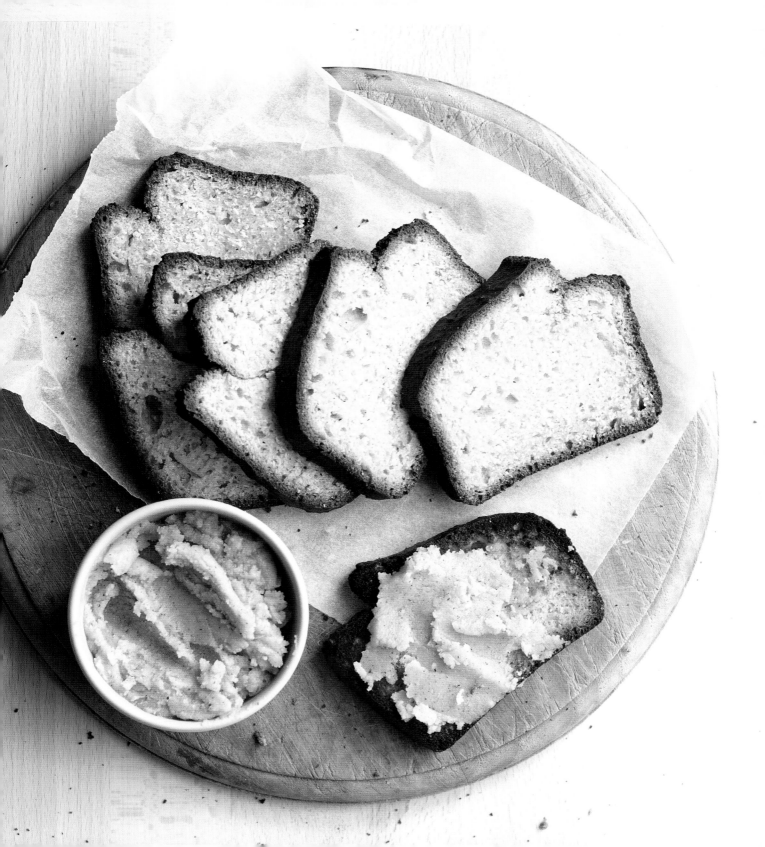

Spelt Soda Bread

makes 1 large loaf

500g (1lb 2oz/4 cups)
wholegrain spelt flour

1 tsp Himalayan pink salt

1 tsp bicarbonate of soda
(baking soda)

25g (1oz) goat's butter

60g (2½oz/scant ⅔ cup) raw
walnuts, chopped

1 egg

300ml (½ pint/scant 1¼ cups)
sheep's yogurt

2–3 tbsp water

This is a great alternative for people on a yeast-free plan and the bicarbonate of soda acts in the same way as yeast, delivering a dense yet light, delicious bread.

Preheat the oven to 220°C/425°F/gas mark 7.

Sift the flour, salt and bicarbonate of soda (baking soda) into a large bowl. Rub in the butter until the mixture resembles fine breadcrumbs, then stir in the walnuts. Whisk the egg into the yogurt and stir into the flour mixture, adding water as necessary to make a soft dough.

Form into a round and place on a greased baking tray (cookie sheet). Bake for 10 minutes, then reduce the heat to 190°C/375°F/gas mark 5 and cook for a further 30–40 minutes, until well risen and the loaf sounds hollow when tapped underneath. Cool on a wire rack.

Sweet Potato Bread

makes 1 small loaf

12.5g (½oz) fresh yeast

150ml (¼ pint/scant ⅔ cup)
warm water

115g (3¾oz/scant 1 cup)
wholegrain spelt flour

100g (3½oz/generous ¾ cup)
rye flour

280g (9¼oz) sweet potato,
grated, squeezed to release
excess juice and patted dry

Sunflower oil, for greasing

You will find sweet potato snuck into a few of our baking recipes as it's such a great healthy 'cheat' to make anything sweet and moist.

Mix the fresh yeast with half the water, cover and set aside in a warm room for about 15 minutes, or until the mixture starts to froth.

Mix the flours and sweet potato in a large bowl, make a well in the centre and add the yeast liquid and remaining water. Mix thoroughly. Turn the dough out onto a lightly floured surface and knead for 10 minutes. Return to the bowl, cover and leave to prove (rise) for 30 minutes in a warm room until almost doubled in size.

Knock back the dough and form into a round loaf. Pop on a greased baking tray (cookie sheet), cover and prove for a further 30 minutes. Meanwhile, preheat the oven to 170°C/340°F/gas mark 3½. Bake the loaf for 40 minutes until well risen. Cool on a wire rack.

Spelt Bread

makes 1 x 500g (1lb) loaf

225g (7½oz/1¾ cups) spelt, rye,
   barley or kamut flour
1 tbsp baking powder
¼ tsp Himalayan pink salt
1 tbsp olive oil
225ml (7½fl oz/scant 1 cup)
   water
1 tbsp date syrup or molasses

If you've given wheat the heave-ho then give this great wheat-free bread a whirl. The mineral content in all these grains is simply superb.

Preheat the oven to 190°C/375°F/gas mark 5.

Mix the dry ingredients in a large bowl. Then, stir the olive oil into the water and stir into the flour. The mixture should be like a thick batter. Transfer to a small loaf tin (19 x 8.5cm/7.5 x 3.5in) and bake for 50–55 minutes, until well risen.

Halfway through baking, brush the top with the molasses or date syrup to give colour to the crust. Turn out onto a wire rack to cool.

Seeded Spelt Bread

makes 1 small loaf

12.5g (½oz) fresh yeast
150ml (½ pint/scant ⅔ cup)
   warm water
115g (3¾oz/scant 1 cup)
   wholegrain spelt flour
100g (3½oz/generous ¾ cup)
   rye flour
½ tsp toasted fennel seeds
½ tsp black onion seeds
½ tsp mustard seeds
Sunflower oil, for greasing

This gorgeously flavoursome bread has the spices hiding in the dough, so is a great accompaniment to any savoury dish.

Mix the fresh yeast with half the water, cover and set aside in a warm room for about 15 minutes, or until the mixture starts to froth.

Mix together the flours and seeds in a large bowl. Make a well in the centre and add the yeast liquid and the remaining water. Mix thoroughly. Turn the dough out onto a lightly floured surface and knead for 10 minutes. Return to the bowl, cover and leave to prove (rise) for 30 minutes until the dough has almost doubled in size.

Knock back the dough and form into a round loaf or break into rolls. Place on a greased baking tray (cookie sheet), cover and prove (rise) for 30 minutes more. Meanwhile, preheat the oven to 170°C/340°F/gas mark 3½. Bake the loaf for 40 minutes, until well risen and the loaf sounds hollow when tapped underneath (rolls will need slightly less time, 25–30 minutes). Cool on a wire rack.

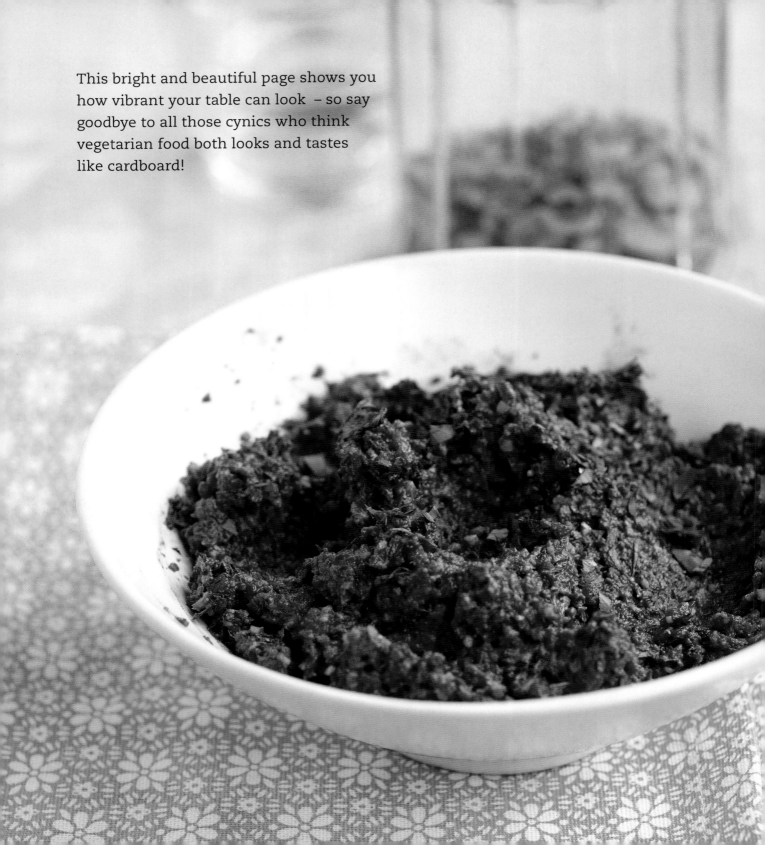

This bright and beautiful page shows you
how vibrant your table can look – so say
goodbye to all those cynics who think
vegetarian food both looks and tastes
like cardboard!

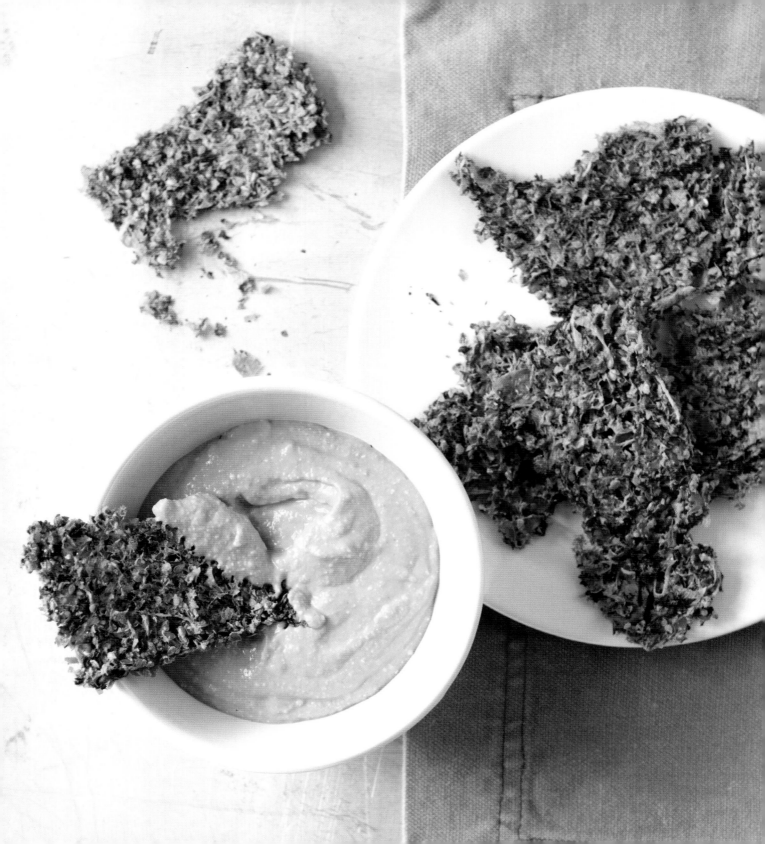

Beetroot and Walnut Dip

serves 3–4

250g (8oz) cooked beetroot (beet), roughly chopped

1–2 garlic cloves, crushed

1 small bunch of coriander (cilantro), roughly chopped

1 small bunch of parsley, roughly chopped

50g (2oz/½ cup) walnuts

3 tsp extra virgin olive oil

2 tsp red wine vinegar

Himalayan pink salt

Freshly ground black pepper

(Pictured on page 164.) The combination of sweet and bitter flavours really whets the palate. Try it as a great afternoon snack or eaten as a mezze or starter.

Place the beetroot (beet), garlic, coriander (cilantro), parsley and walnuts in a food processor and whizz to a coarse paste. Transfer the mixture to a bowl, add the olive oil and red wine vinegar, season with salt and pepper, and stir to combine.

Serve with crudités or as part of a salad.

Smoky Aubergine Dip

serves 3–4

2 large aubergines (eggplant)

20g (¾oz) tahini

2 garlic cloves

Juice of 1 lemon

Olive oil, to garnish

Sumac, to garnish

Bread or crudités, to serve

To create this dip's wonderful smoky taste, cook the aubergines (eggplant) over a naked flame, over a medium heat on the hob, on a barbecue or in a very hot oven. The smell of the skin burning is exactly what you want.

Cook the aubergines (eggplant) for about 5 minutes, until very soft, turning frequently. When the aubergines (eggplant) are cool enough to handle, rip off the stalks and peel away the skin.

Whizz the aubergine (eggplant) flesh in a blender with the tahini, garlic and lemon juice until smooth.

Serve in a bowl garnished with a swirl of olive oil and a sprinkle of sumac accompanied with wheat-free bread or crudités.

NUTRITIONAL NUGGET
Garlic supports liver function, and tahini is a rich source of the antioxidant selenium, as well as being a vegetarian protein.

Raw Flax Seed Crackers

makes 10 crackers

♥♥♥ 🌱

185g (6½oz) carrots, roughly chopped

250g (8oz) tomatoes, roughly chopped

20g (¾oz) coriander (cilantro)

80ml (3fl oz/⅓ cup) water

10g (½oz) spring onion (scallion), finely chopped

Juice of ½ lemon

Pinch of Himalayan pink salt

Pinch of ground cumin

20g (¾oz/generous ⅛ cup) raw flax seeds, soaked for 2 hours

(Pictured on page 165.) Imagine sitting in Italy and smelling the aromas of all the local foods – well, this über-healthy cracker tastes like a Mediterranean scene and just fills your taste buds with love!

Blend the carrots, tomatoes and coriander (cilantro) with the water to a rough pulp, then transfer to a strainer and drain well. Place in a mixing bowl and add the spring onion (scallion), lemon juice and a pinch each of salt and cumin. Drain the flax seeds, squeezing out as much liquid as possible with the back of a wooden spoon. Add them to the rest of the ingredients and stir well to combine.

Spread the mixture out on a dehydrator sheet to a thickness of 2cm (¾in) – it will shrink! Place in the dehydrator and dehydrate for 10 hours (see also page 54). Break into crackers when dried.

Spinach and Chickpea Hummus

serves 4

♥♥♥ 🌱

400g (13oz/2 cups) canned chickpeas, rinsed and drained

60g (2½oz) spinach

1 tbsp tahini

Juice of ½ lemon

2 tbsp olive oil

1 small garlic clove

About 125ml (4fl oz/½ cup) water

(Pictured on page 165.) Chickpeas are the perfect base for any flavour or seasoning. I love the colour the spinach adds to this yummy dip.

Place the chickpeas, spinach, tahini, lemon juice and olive oil in a blender, grate in the garlic clove and whizz to a paste, gradually adding the water until it forms the consistency you like.

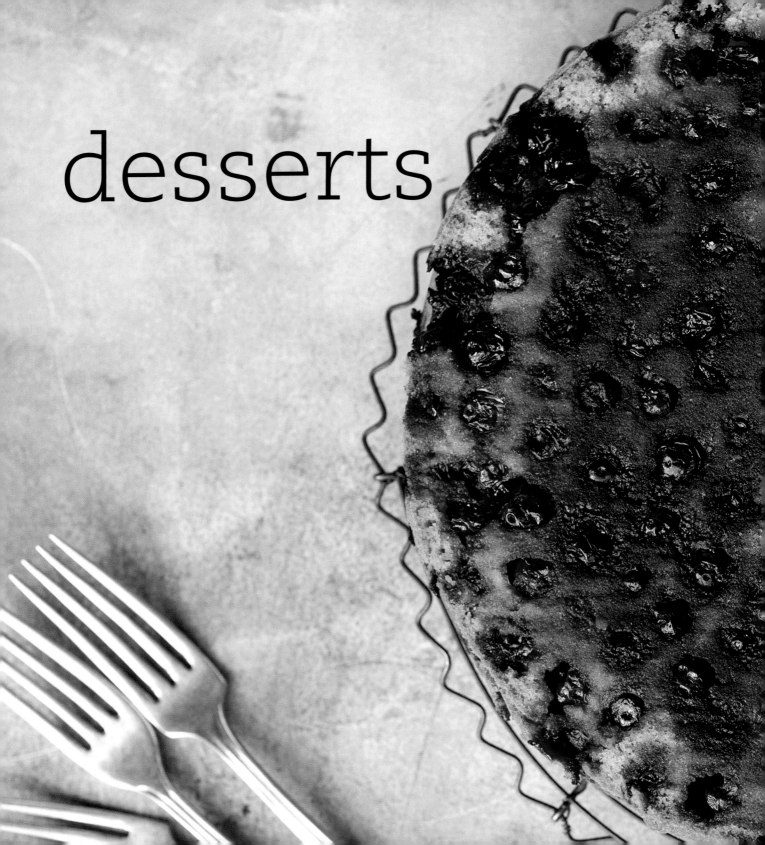

desserts

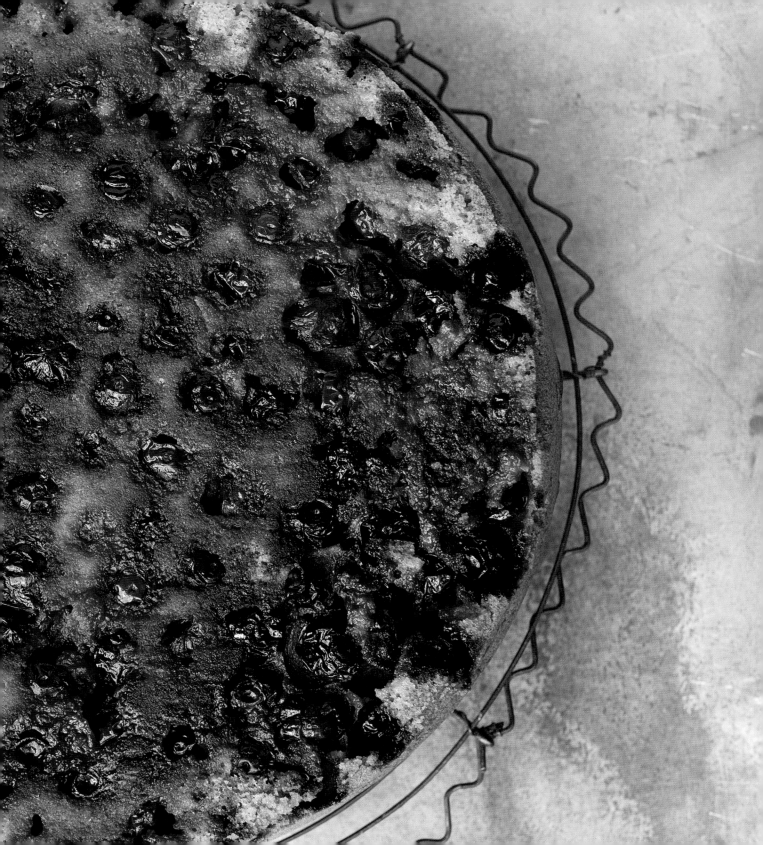

Blueberry Polenta Cake

serves 10

300g (10oz/2 cups) blueberries
4 large eggs
200g (7oz) xylitol
1½ tsp vanilla extract
Seeds from ¼ vanilla pod
  (vanilla bean)
250ml (8fl oz/1 cup) sunflower
  oil, plus extra for greasing
250ml (8fl oz/1 cup) apple juice
250g (8oz/2 cups) white spelt
  flour
110g (3¾oz/scant ⅔ cup) fine
  polenta (cornmeal)
1 tsp baking powder

(Pictured on pages 168–169). This is a show-stopper of a cake! The colour of the blueberries when they have burst on the surface is irresistible. Serve with some raw vanilla ice cream and you have a perfect indulgence.

Preheat the oven to 180°C/350°F/gas mark 4. Place the blueberries in the bottom of a greased 23cm (9in) springform cake tin, base-lined with baking parchment.

Beat the eggs with the xylitol and the vanilla extract and seeds until foamy. Beat in the oil, then the apple juice. Sift in the flour, polenta (cornmeal) and baking powder, then fold in, making sure there are no lumps. Pour the batter into the cake tin and bake for 1½ hours, or until a skewer inserted into the cake comes out clean.

Leave to cool in the tin, then release the side of the tin, place a serving plate over the cake and quickly flip it over so the blueberries are now on the top. Very carefully remove the baking parchment.

Raw Chocolate Mousse

serves 2

1 tbsp coconut oil
1 avocado
1 tsp water
2 heaped tbsp raw cacao
  powder
2 tbsp agave syrup (or more, to
  taste)
Raspberries or blackberries,
  to serve

Try this fun party game – ask your guests what unexpected green ingredient they think is in this velvety mousse. They will never guess!

Melt the coconut oil in a heatproof bowl set over a pan of hot water, then transfer to a blender with the avocado flesh and water and whizz until very smooth. Add the cacao powder and agave syrup or honey and whizz again until completely smooth. Taste and add a little more agave syrup, if required.

Put the mousse in a dish for two or, if you prefer, divide the mixture between 2 ramekins. Chill in the refrigerator for at least 1 hour.

Serve with raspberries or blackberries... delish!

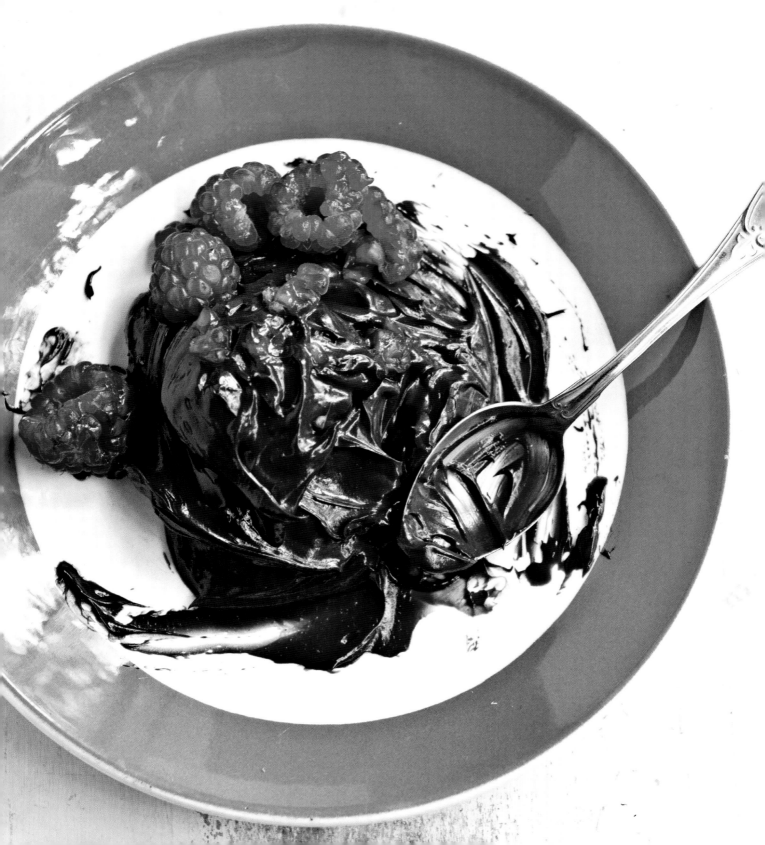

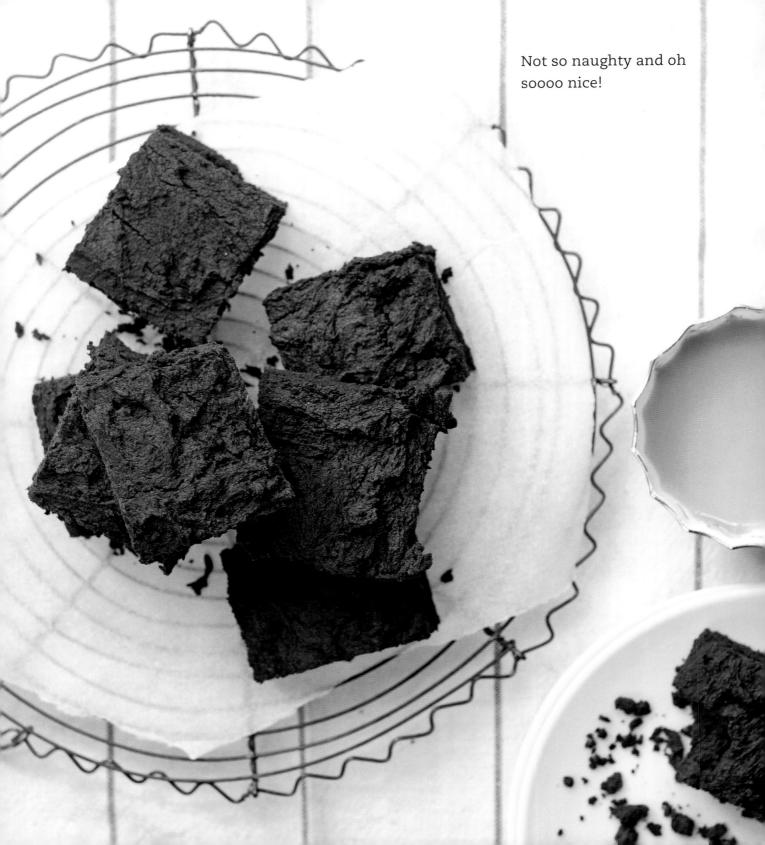

Not so naughty and oh soooo nice!

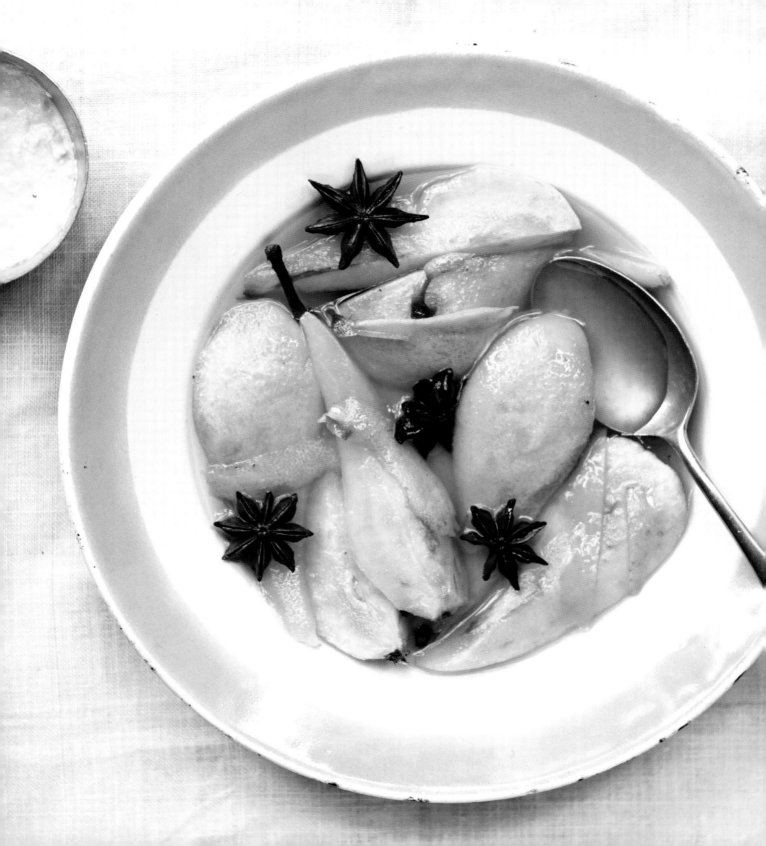

Sweet-Potato Chocolate Brownies

makes 8

125g (4oz/generous ¾ cup) rice flour

75g (3oz/¾ cup) raw cacao powder

¼ tsp baking powder

175g (6oz) sweet potato, cooked and mashed to a purée

250g (8oz/scant ¾ cup) date syrup

175g (6oz/scant ¾ cup) goat's butter, melted

1 egg

¼ tsp vanilla extract

(Pictured on page 172.) In trying to create the perfect healthy brownie, moisture was definitely an issue. Our secret ingredient? The sweet potato – our saving grace.

Preheat the oven to 180°C/350°F/gas mark 4.

Sift the rice flour, cacao powder and baking powder into a bowl.

Place the sweet potato purée, date syrup, melted butter, egg and vanilla extract in another bowl and mix together well. Then stir in the dry ingredients.

Pour the brownie mixture into a rectangular cake tin lined with baking parchment and bake for 20–25 minutes, until set on top but gooey in the middle.

Cool in the tin, then cut into 8 pieces.

WHAT IS RAW CACAO POWDER?
This is one of the most amazing 'superfoods'. It's so rich in antioxidants, which help to make our systems strong to fight of any illnesses.

Poached Pears with Star Anise and Cashew Cream

serves 4

4 ripe firm pears, peeled,
   quartered and cored
5 star anise
30g (1¼oz) agave syrup
150g (5oz/1 cup) raw cashews
½ tsp vanilla extract

(Pictured on page 173.) A perfect quick and easy sweet fix and after-dinner treat, particularly for those who want to clear their palate after a meal.

Preheat the oven to 160°C/325°F/gas mark 3.

Place the pear quarters in an ovenproof dish large enough to hold them without overlapping, add water to half cover the pears, then add the star anise and drizzle over 2 teaspoons of the agave syrup. Bake for about 25 minutes, or until tender.

Meanwhile, whizz the cashews with the vanilla extract and 225ml (7½fl oz/scant 1 cup) of water in a blender until smooth and creamy. Transfer to a serving bowl.

When the pears are cooked, remove them from the dish with a slotted spoon and set aside. Pour half the cooking liquid into a pan with 2 of the star anise and the remaining agave syrup and place over a high heat for about 5 minutes, stirring constantly, until the liquid becomes thick and syrupy.

Serve the pears with the syrup, cashew cream and a little of the remaining cooking liquid.

Chocolate Superfood Ganache

serves 12–14

For the chocolate sauce

400g (13oz/4 cups) raw cacao
   powder
2 tsp cinnamon
950ml (1²/₃ pints/3²/₃ cups)
   agave syrup
2 tsp Himalayan pink salt
2 tsp vanilla extract
125g (4oz/½ cup) coconut oil

For the ganache

1 quantity of Chocolate Sauce
3 tbsp maca powder
1 tbsp spirulina
1 tsp cinnamon
75g (3oz/scant ²/₃ cup) shelled
   raw hemp seeds

NUTRITIONAL NUGGET

Hemp seeds are packed
with the essential fatty acids
omega-3 and omega-6 oils
in one of the healthiest ratios
around. What's more, these
seed are a rich source of
the super-polyunsaturated
fatty acids, notably gamma-
linolenic acid.

This is the most rich and indulgent recipe in the whole
book. Enjoy with no guilt at all, as you deserve it – and
anyway, it's full of superfoods!

To make the sauce, whizz the ingredients in a blender until smooth.

To make the ganache, whizz the chocolate sauce with the maca
powder, spirulina and cinnamon in a blender until smooth. Pour into
a 20cm (8in) square baking tin or springform cake tin, lined with
baking parchment, and sprinkle over the shelled hemp seeds.

Place the tin in the freezer for 20 minutes until the ganache is set,
then cut into portions and enjoy.

WHAT IS RAW MACA POWDER?

Maca is a food the Incan gods considered an aphrodisiac. Some say this
fantastic antioxidant helps to regulate hormones. Deliciously sweet, it's
excellent in baking. It should be avoided by anyone with breast cancer.

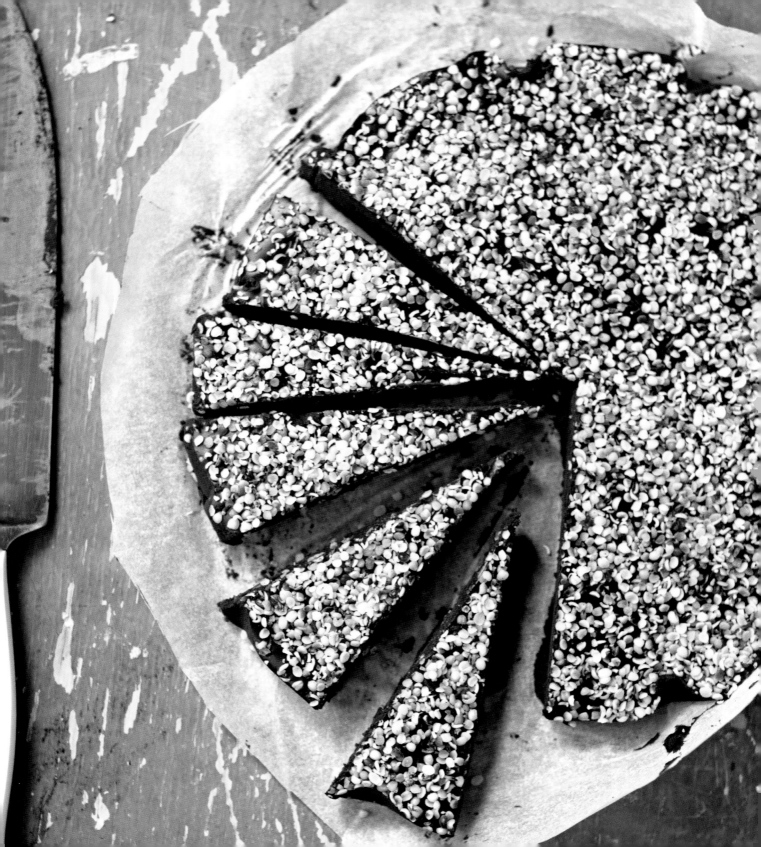

Lemon and Poppy Seed Almond Cake

serves 10

4 eggs

60g (2½oz/scant ¼ cup) honey

200g (7oz/generous ¾ cup) vegan butter, plus extra for greasing

250g (8oz/2 cups) ground almonds

1 tsp baking powder

Finely grated zest and juice of 3 small or 2 large lemons

2 tbsp poppy seeds

Melted raw chocolate, for topping (optional)

This is quite simply my favourite cake ever – it's so easy and quick to make. Just pop on a few candles and, hey presto, you have a perfect birthday cake.

Preheat the oven to 160°C/325°F/gas mark 3.

Whisk the eggs and honey together in a bowl.

Mix the butter and ground almonds thoroughly in a separate bowl, then gradually stir in the egg mixture until smooth.

Add the baking powder and the lemon zest and juice and mix thoroughly, then stir in the poppy seeds.

Pour the mixture into a greased 20–25cm (8–10in) springform cake tin and bake for 30 minutes, until golden (cover the top with foil if it starts to brown too quickly). The cake is cooked when the top feels springy when you press it gently, or the tip of a sharp knife or skewer inserted into the centre of the cake comes out clean.

Cool on a wire rack, then top with melted chocolate, if using.

TIPS

Some extra special tweaks:

- Omit the poppy seeds and use the finely grated zest of 2 small oranges instead of the lemons for an orange almond cake.
- Omit the poppy seeds, add 50g (2oz/½ cup) raw cacao powder and reduce the almonds to 200g (7oz/scant 1⅔ cups) for a chocolatey one.

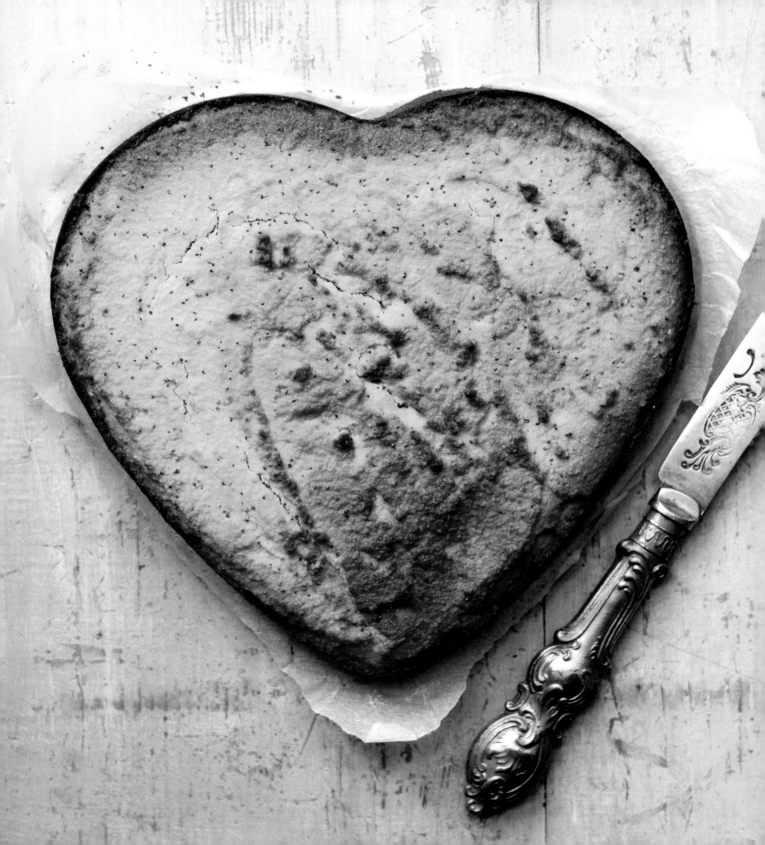

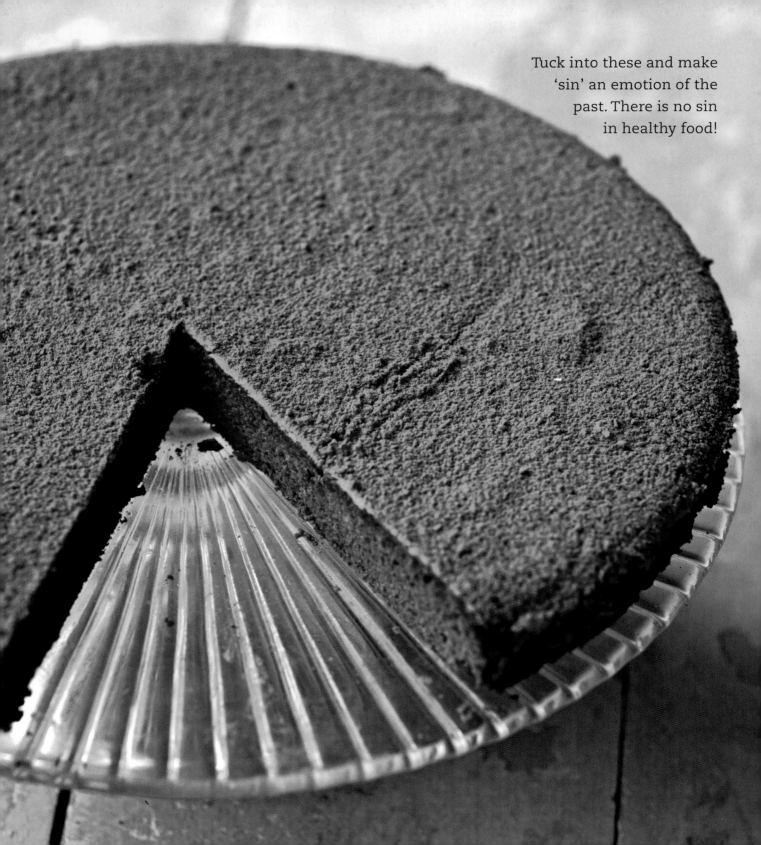

Tuck into these and make 'sin' an emotion of the past. There is no sin in healthy food!

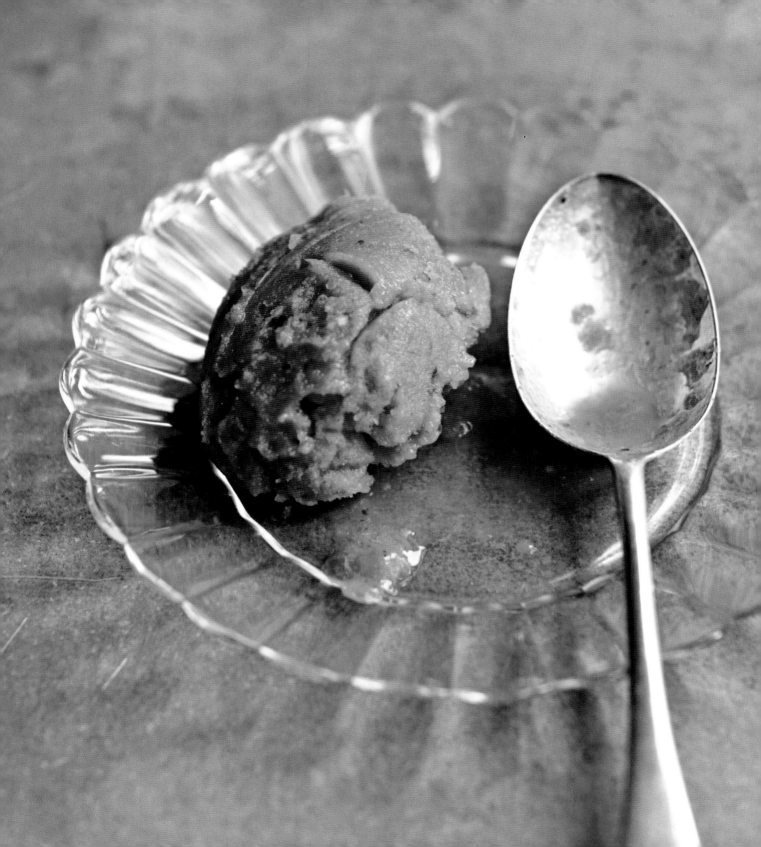

Coconut Flour Chocolate Mousse Cake

serves 10–12

100g (3½oz/generous ¾ cup)
  coconut flour
50g (2oz/½ cup) raw cacao
  powder, plus ½ tbsp for
  dusting
500ml (17fl oz/2 cups) Hemp
  Milk (see page 57)
120g (4oz/½ cup) light olive oil
  non-dairy spread, plus extra
  for greasing
130g (4¼oz/⅓ cup) agave syrup
2 tbsp yacon syrup
2 tbsp almond butter
4 eggs
1 tsp vanilla extract

(Pictured on page 180.) This is a very dense, moist cake and is too amazing for words! Either make a thin 'torte', as illustrated here, or bake in a smaller tin for a deeper, more luxurious-looking cake.

Preheat the oven to 150°C/300°F/gas mark 2.

Sift the coconut flour and cacao powder into a bowl.

Place the hemp milk, dairy-free margarine, syrups, almond butter, eggs and vanilla essence (vanilla extract) in a blender and whizz for about 1 minute, until well blended (the mixture will be a little frothy on top). Gently fold the wet ingredients into the flour mixture until combined. The mixture will have quite a thick consistency.

Transfer the mixture to a lightly greased, base-lined springform cake tin (use a large, shallow tin for a thin, torte-like cake or a smaller, deeper tin for a thicker cake). Bake for 30–50 minutes, depending on the thickness. The thicker the cake, the longer it will need – check after 30 minutes by inserting a skewer into the centre of the cake. If it comes out clean, then it is cooked. Otherwise, continue cooking, checking every 10 minutes. The cake will continue to set when cooling.

Leave to cool in the tin for 30 minutes, then transfer to a serving plate. Serve warm or cold, lightly dusted with cacao powder, with a scoop of one of our ice creams or sorbets (see pages 183–189).

WHAT IS YACON SYRUP?
This dark, thick caramel-like syrup is a sugar alternative. It's packed with fructo-oligosaccharides, which are sugars that aid digestion and which are absorbed slowly into the bloodstream, as well as being high in vitamins A, C and E.

Lychee, Mango and Basil Sorbet

serves 4–6

200g (7oz) lychees, peeled and pitted

200g (7oz) mango, chopped

1 tsp grated lime zest

2 tbsp lime juice

150ml (5fl oz/scant ⅔ cup) agave syrup

225ml (7½fl oz/scant 1 cup) water

3 packed tbsp basil leaves

(Pictured on page 181.) This will blow the socks off any sorbet you have tried – you don't need lashings of sugar, as you'll see, to make this a wonderfully sweet fix.

Whizz all the ingredients in a blender until smooth.

Transfer the mixture to an ice-cream maker and freeze according to the manufacturer's instructions. Transfer to a freezer-proof container, cover and freeze until firm.

If you don't have an ice-cream maker, transfer the mixture to a shallow freezer-proof dish and place in the freezer until it just starts to harden around the edges. Whisk vigorously with a fork to break up any ice crystals, then freeze until firm.

NUTRITIONAL NUGGET
Basil has abundant vitamin C and its essential oil is highly protective for the skin. This could explain why it is native to hot countries – nature will always provide what is needed, where it's needed.

Shepherd's Chocolate Ice Cream

serves 6–8

350ml (12fl oz/1⅓ cups) goat's milk

150g (5oz) xylitol

3 large egg yolks

475ml (16fl oz/scant 2 cups) sheep's yogurt

1 tsp vanilla essence (vanilla extract)

½ tsp vanilla powder

3 tbsp raw cacao powder

1 tbsp mesquite powder

2 tbsp raw cacao butter, melted

WHAT IS XYLITOL?
Xylitol has the lowest glycaemic index (GI) of all the sugar alternatives. It's super-sweet but has a fresh minty undertone (why it's used in chewing gum) and is also rumoured to be good for your teeth. It's great for baking!

We call it 'shepherd's' ice cream because it's made with sheep's yogurt, which just makes it feel incredibly indulgent and creamy beyond belief. So, enjoy your chocolate ice cream – 'cos you can!

Combine the goat's milk and 100g (3½oz) of the xylitol in a heavy pan and bring to a simmer, stirring constantly, until the xylitol starts to dissolve.

Whisk the egg yolks with the remaining xylitol in a large, heatproof bowl until blended. Gradually add the hot milk mixture, whisking constantly, until blended. Return the mixture to the pan and cook, stirring constantly, over a medium-low heat for about 3 minutes, or until the custard thickens slightly and coats the back of the spoon. Be careful not to let it boil. Remove from the heat and set aside to cool, stirring occasionally to make sure it doesn't split.

Meanwhile, combine the yogurt, vanilla essence (vanilla extract) and vanilla powder in a large bowl. Gradually whisk the cooled custard into the yogurt mixture.

Stir the cacao powder and mesquite powder into the melted cacao butter and gently whisk into the custard mixture.

Transfer the mixture to an ice-cream maker and freeze according to the manufacturer's instructions. Transfer to a freezer-proof container, cover and freeze until firm.

If you don't have an ice-cream maker, transfer the mixture to a shallow freezer-proof dish and place in the freezer until it just starts to harden around the edges. Whisk vigorously with a fork to break up any ice crystals, then freeze until firm.

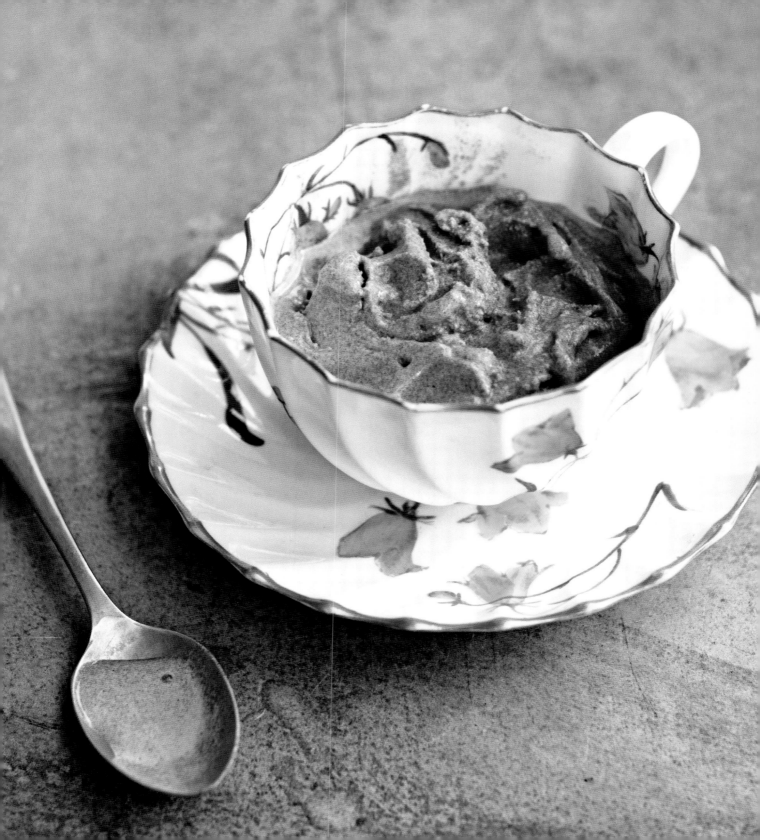

Banana Toffee Crunch Ice Cream

serves 4–6

225ml (7½fl oz/scant 1 cup)
   Almond Milk (see page 57)
200g (7oz) xylitol
475ml (16fl oz/scant 2 cups)
   sheep's yogurt
¼ tsp xanthan gum
1½ tbsp agave syrup
1½ tsp lemon juice
2 bananas, chopped

For the toffee brittle
1 tsp coconut oil, melted
4 tbsp Brazil nut butter
1 tsp agave syrup
50g (2oz/generous ⅓ cup) raw
   pecans, chopped
3 fresh dates, pitted and
   chopped
Pinch of Himalayan pink salt

This is toffee without the toffee. It's a little more complicated to make but is definitely worth having a go, and the end result is a match for any Italian ice cream.

To make the toffee brittle, stir all the ingredients together in a bowl, then spread onto a flat baking tray (cookie sheet), cover with cling film and freeze for about 40 minutes, until hard.

Combine the almond milk and xylitol in a pan and bring to a simmer, stirring constantly, until the xylitol starts to dissolve. Allow to cool, then gradually whisk into the yogurt in a bowl, adding the xanthan gum halfway through.

Stir in the agave syrup and lemon juice and finally add the bananas.

Transfer the mixture to an ice-cream maker and freeze according to the manufacturer's instructions. Transfer to a freezer-proof container, cover and freeze until firm, adding the toffee brittle, broken into small pieces, once the ice cream is set but not too firm.

If you don't have an ice-cream maker, transfer the mixture to a shallow freezer-proof dish and place in the freezer until it just starts to harden around the edges. Whisk vigorously with a fork to break up any ice crystals, then freeze until firm.

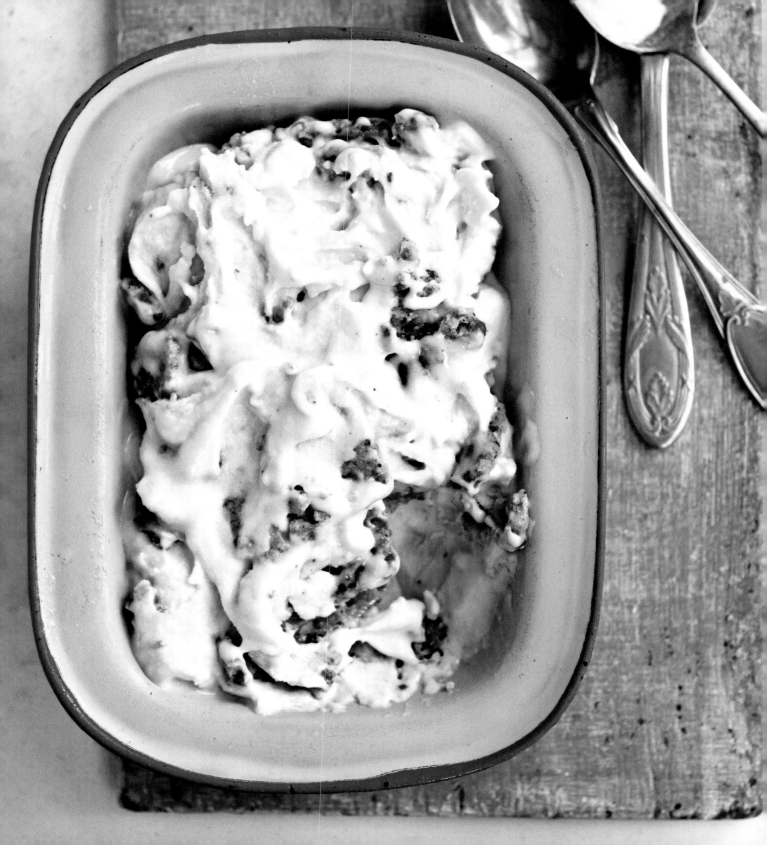

Strawberry and Coconut Ice Cream

serves 4

250g (8oz/2 cups) strawberries

225ml (7½fl oz/scant 1 cup) coconut cream

125ml (4fl oz/½ cup) coconut water

2 tbsp agave syrup

¼ tsp vanilla powder

½ tsp xanthan gum

½ tsp lemon juice

Making ice cream doesn't have to be a tricky game – it takes a little patience, but this recipe is very easy and the chunks of strawberry give it such a great vibrancy.

Chop and gently crush 50g (2oz/generous ⅓ cup) of the strawberries and set aside.

Whizz the remaining ingredients in a blender until smooth. Decant the mixture into a bowl and stir in the crushed strawberries. Transfer to an ice-cream maker and freeze according to the manufacturer's instructions. Put in a freezer-proof container, cover and freeze until firm.

If you don't have an ice-cream maker, transfer the mixture to a shallow freezer-proof dish and place in the freezer until it just starts to harden around the edges. Whisk vigorously with a fork to break up any ice crystals, then freeze until firm.

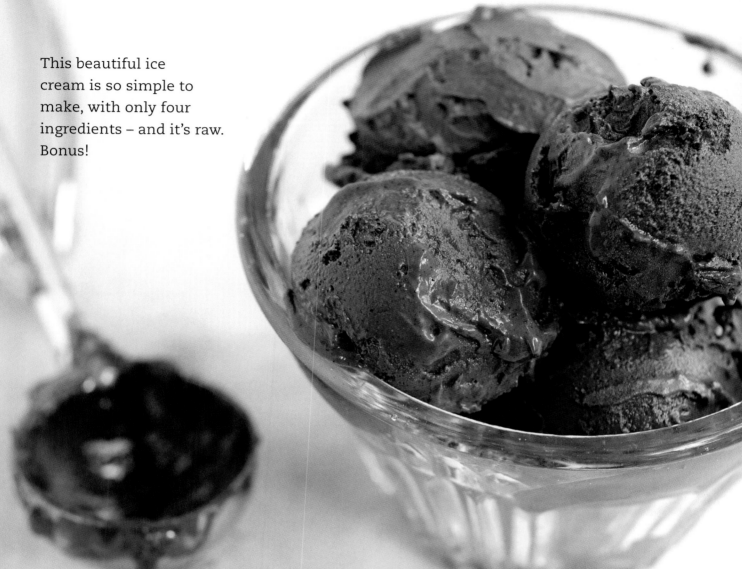

This beautiful ice cream is so simple to make, with only four ingredients – and it's raw. Bonus!

Raw Blueberry Ice Cream

serves 4

100g (3½oz/⅔ cup) raw cashews
180g (6oz/generous 1⅛ cups)
   frozen blueberries
80ml (3fl oz/⅓ cup) water
2 tbsp agave syrup

Whizz all the ingredients in a blender until smooth, then freeze in an ice-cream maker according to the manufacturer's instructions. Transfer to a freezer-proof container, cover and freeze until firm.

If you don't have an ice-cream maker, transfer the mixture to a shallow freezer-proof dish and place in the freezer until it just starts to harden around the edges. Whisk vigorously with a fork to break up any ice crystals, then freeze until firm.

Index

Big Thank Yous from Tash and Vix

We would like to give a huge thank you to Jacqui Small for making the book happen and seeing our vision. To Lisa Linder, with her amazing photographic skills made our food look as utterly mouthwatering as it tastes. And to the book's whole team for their perseverance, patience and politeness. Thank you to Kelly (Mummy) for letting me steal (without knowing) most of her crockery and cutlery for the shoot! Big love to the British farmers and growers who have provided us with the most delicious produce for us to create with.

Tash says: I would like to send massive healthy love to Hayley North for being involved in this book. I'd like to thank all my friends for being such great guinea pigs, by making all the right noises at my dinners. A huge loving thank you to my dad for sitting in the 'cupboard' on skype talking to me when I was cooking at home alone. The two wonderful fruit & veg stalls outside number 158 Portobello Road for their ever-tasty veg and letting us do our photo shoot. And a grateful hug to Joshi who introduced me to how amazing alkaline living can really be.

Vix says: To Robert Young, the pioneer of the alkaline approach who I had the good fortune to meet several years ago, and whose radiance and total focus inspired me. To my many clients who have given me feedback on the principles of the Cleanse and Lifestyle and shown me the results! And to Mother Nature herself who always provides us with what we need to sustain and nourish ourselves.

Directory of Food Suppliers

At Honestly Healthy, we source everything we can from London-based stores. Our favourites are:

Planet Organic, which has five stores across London and an online shop. www.planetorganic.com

Portobello Wholefoods on Portobello Road. If you are local, you'll probably know it already; if not, take a trip to come see this fabulous treasure trove of a store at 266 Portobello Road, London W10 5TY.

You can buy pretty much everything in one place at **Infinity Foods** online shop; they have a bricks-and-mortar shop, too, in Brighton. www.infinityfoods.co.uk

I buy lots of our super-foods from **www.guaranaco.com**

There are lots of suppliers online and you'll no doubt find your own favourites; here's a list to start you off.

You can find pretty much everything you need at **WholeFoods Market**. They have six stores in the UK, seven in Canada, and full US state coverage. www.wholefoodsmarket.com

For fantastic omega oil supplements, check out **www.udoschoice.co.uk**

A great American-based store **www.sunwarrior.com**

Get all sorts of super-foods at **www.detoxyourworld.com**

For British-grown hemp products go to **Good Oil** www.goodwebsite.co.uk

Buy seeds to sprout from **Living Food of St Ives** www.livingfood.co.uk

Or buy them ready-sprouted from **Aconbury Sprouts** at www.wheatgrass-uk.com

Steenberg's Organic do a great spice selection, as well as other foodstuffs www.steenbergs.co.uk

You can buy pretty much everything you need at **www.buywholefoodsonline.co.uk**

Pukka Herbs has stores all over the world including the US and Australia. www.pukkaherbs.com

A wide range of organic foodstuffs can be found at **www.organicsaustraliaonline.com.au**

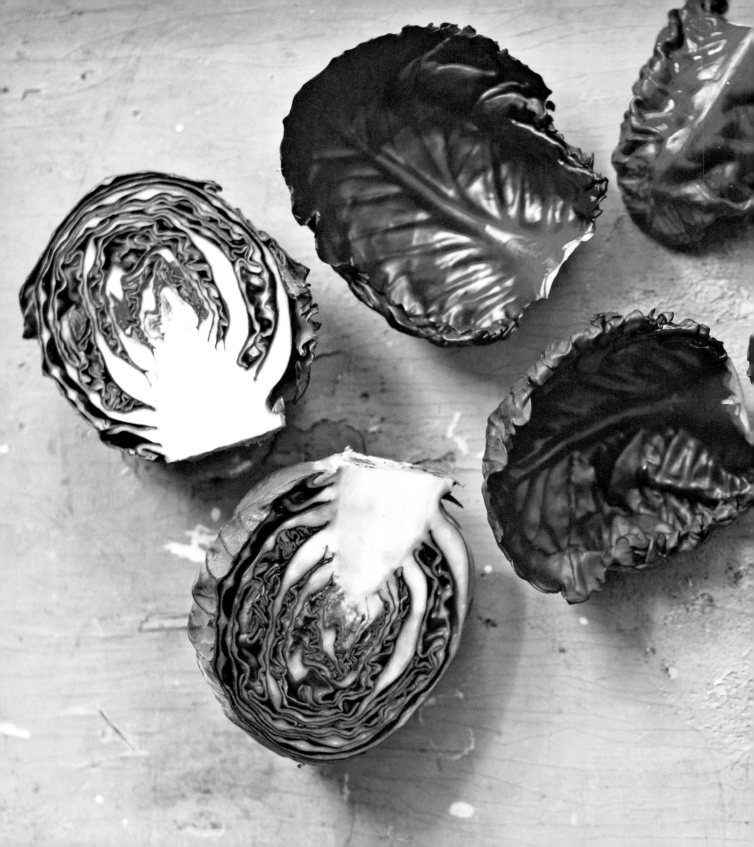